W9-CKQ-633

Wound Care

made Incredibly Visual!

Third Edition

Wound Care

made Incredibly Visual!

Third Edition

Clinical Editor

Patricia Albano Slachta, PhD, APRN, ACNS-BC, CWOCN

President, Nursing Educational Programs & Services
State College, Pennsylvania

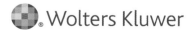 Wolters Kluwer

Philadelphia • Baltimore • New York • London
Buenos Aires • Hong Kong • Sydney • Tokyo

Executive Editor: Nicole Dernoski
Development Editor: Maria M. McAvey
Editorial Coordinator: Kayla Smull
Production Project Manager: Barton Dudlick
Design Coordinator: Elaine Kasmer
Manufacturing Coordinator: Kathleen Brown
Marketing Manager: Linda Wetmore
Prepress Vendor: SPi Global

3rd Edition

Library of Congress Cataloging-in-Publication Data
Names: Slachta, Patricia A., editor.
Title: Wound care made incredibly visual / clinical editor, Patricia Albano Slachta.
Description: 3rd edition. | Philadelphia : Wolters Kluwer, [2019] | Includes bibliographical references and index.
Identifiers: LCCN 2018034658 | ISBN 9781496398260 (paperback)
Subjects: | MESH: Wounds and Injuries—nursing | Handbooks | Atlases
Classification: LCC RD93.95 | NLM WY 49 | DDC 617.1—dc23 LC record available at https://lccn.loc.gov/2018034658

Dedication

To my husband Greg, daughters Jennifer and Andrea, and my grandchildren Brendan, Cooper, Alexander, Ethan, Abby, Kelyn and Addie for their continuing love and support throughout my career. I love you all and could not do it without you.

Patricia Albano Slachta

Contributors

Carol Calianno, MSN, CWOCN, CRNP
Nurse/Practitioner
Dermatology/Wound Care
CMC Veteran's Medical Center
Philadelphia, Pennsylvania

Anne Elizabeth Johnson, MSN, RN, CWON
Professional Education Manager
Fort Worth, Texas

Lynette E. Franklin, APRN, ACNS-BC,
    CWOCN-AP, CFCN
Clinical Nurse Specialist, APRN
The Emory Clinic
Atlanta, Georgia

Teresa J. Kelechi, PhD, RN, GCNS, CWCN, FAAN
David and Margaret Clare Endowed Chair
College of Nursing
Medical University of South Carolina
Charleston, South Carolina

Kathy McLaughlin, DNP, RN, CWOCN
Wound, Ostomy and Continence Nursing
Paoli Hospital
Paoli, Pennsylvania

Jody N. Scardillo, DNP, RN, ANP-BC, CWOCN
Clinical Nurse Specialist/Nurse
    Practitioner
WOC Nursing
Albany Medical Center
Albany, New York

Charleen Singh, PhD, FNP-BC, CWOCN, RN
Nurse Practitioner
General Surgery
Cottage Hospital
Santa Barbara, California

Previous Edition Contributors

Debbie Berry, RN, MSN, CPHQ, CWCN, CCCN

Laura A. Conklin, RN, MSN, MSA, ONC, CWS,
LNCC, FCCWS, DIP. AAWM

Evonne Fowler, RN, CWON

Elizabeth R. Fudge, RN, MS, CWON

Julia Isen, RN, MS, FNP-C

Jennifer L. Pettis, RN, WCC, RAC-MT

Michelle C. Quigel, RN, BSN, CWOCN

Tracy A. Robinson, RN, BSN, CWOCN

Tracey J. Siegel, MSN, RN, CWOCN, CNE

Jennifer Smoltz, RN, MSN, CWOCN, ACNP-BC

Acknowledgment

In appreciation to:

Mandy Spitzer, BSN, RN, CWOCN, CFCN, who provided her expertise during the revision of this book.

My many wound care colleagues who inspire nurses and physicians to provide patients with excellent wound care every day.

Patricia

Contents

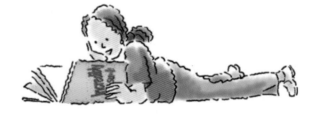

Chapter 1

Skin anatomy and physiology

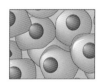

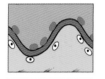
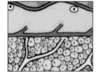

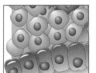
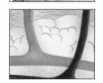
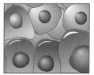
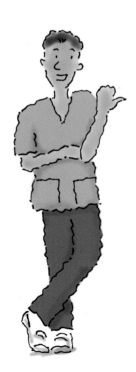

Anatomy

The skin, or integumentary system, is the largest organ in the body. It accounts for 6 to 8 lb (2.5 to 3.5 kg) of a person's body weight and is reflective of the person's surface area. In some cases, the surface area is more than 20 square feet. The skin's composition includes living and nonliving cells. The living cells in the skin receive oxygen and nutrients through an extensive network of small blood vessels.

Collaboration is key. The skin is made up of two separate layers, which consist of unique sublayers that function as a single unit. A third layer, the subcutaneous tissue or hypodermis, sits just below the dermis.

Cross section of the skin

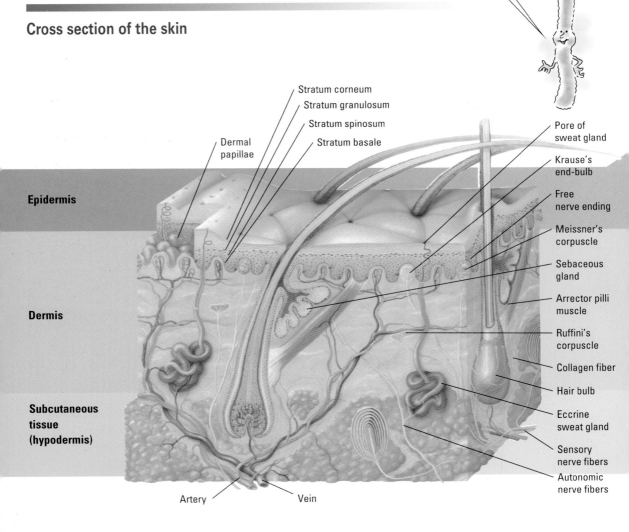

Stratum corneum
Stratum granulosum
Stratum spinosum
Stratum basale
Dermal papillae
Pore of sweat gland
Krause's end-bulb
Free nerve ending
Meissner's corpuscle
Sebaceous gland
Arrector pili muscle
Ruffini's corpuscle
Collagen fiber
Hair bulb
Eccrine sweat gland
Sensory nerve fibers
Autonomic nerve fibers
Epidermis
Dermis
Subcutaneous tissue (hypodermis)
Artery
Vein

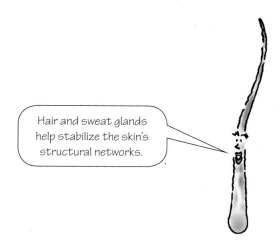

Hair and sweat glands help stabilize the skin's structural networks.

Functions of the skin layers

Layer	Description
Epidermis	• Outermost layer • Consists of five sublayers • Formed mainly by keratinocytes (cells that are continuously generated and migrate from the underlying dermis and die upon reaching the surface) • Contains melanocytes (give skin and hair their color), Langerhans cells (provide the skin with immunological function), and Merkel's cells (serve as markers of tactile function; confined to the lips and fingertips) • Regenerates itself every 4 to 6 weeks • Serves as a protective layer against water loss and physical damage
Dermis	• Composed of collagen fibers (give skin its strength), elastin fibers (provide elasticity), and an extracellular matrix (contributes to skin's strength and pliability) • Consists of two sublayers: the papillary dermis (outer layer composed of collagen and reticular fibers) and the reticular dermis (inner layer formed by thick networks of collagen bundles that anchor onto subcutaneous tissue and underlying support structures) • Contains blood and lymphatic vessels (supply nutrition and remove wastes), nerve fibers, hair follicles, sebaceous and sweat glands, and fibroblast cells (important in the production of collagen and elastin) • Supplies nutrition to the skin and supports the skin's structure and strength
Subcutaneous tissue (hypodermis)	• Subdermal layer of adipose and connective tissue • Contains major blood vessels, lymph vessels, and nerves • Insulates the body, absorbs shocks to the skeletal system, and helps skin move easily over underlying structures • Varies in thickness based on person's habitus

A closer look at epidermal layers

The epidermis consists of five distinct layers. The innermost layer contains protrusions (called *rete pegs* or *epidermal ridges*) that extend down into the dermis. Surrounded by vascularized dermal papillae, these protrusions support the epidermis and facilitate the exchange of fluids and cells between skin layers.

> Let me get this straight: the skin has two main layers and a third layer that sits just below the dermis. Of those three layers, the outermost layer has five layers of its own, the second layer has two layers, and the final deeper layer varies in thickness based on the person's habitus. If that were a cake, I'd need a lot of icing.

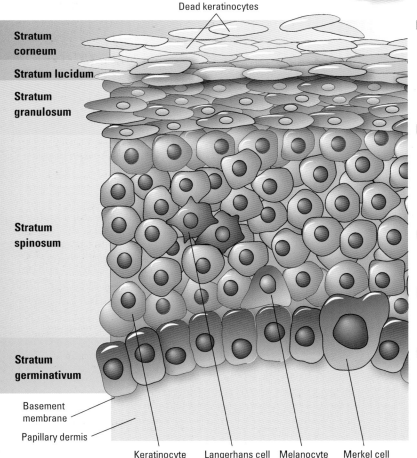

Dead keratinocytes

Stratum corneum

Stratum lucidum

Stratum granulosum

Stratum spinosum

Stratum germinativum

Basement membrane

Papillary dermis

Keratinocyte   Langerhans cell   Melanocyte   Merkel cell

The stratum corneum (a superficial layer of dead skin cells—corneocytes) has contact with the environment. The cells here shed daily and are replaced with cells from the layer beneath it (keratinocytes).

The stratum lucidum (a single layer of cells) is most evident in areas where skin is thick—such as the palms and soles—and appears to be absent where skin is especially thin—such as the eyelids.

The stratum granulosum (one to five cells thick) aids keratin formation and lamellated granules.

The stratum spinosum is where cells begin to flatten as they migrate toward the skin surface.

The stratum germinativum, or stratum basale, is one cell thick and is the only layer in which cells undergo mitosis to form new cells. This layer also contains melanocytes and Merkel's cells.

A closer look at the dermis

The dermis is considered the living layer of the skin with rich blood supply, nerve endings, sebaceous glands, and hair follicles. The dermal layer is thicker in comparison to the epidermis layer and contributes to skin turgor. Collagen and elastin within the dermal layer gives skin its tensile strength.

Blood supply

The skin receives its blood supply through vessels that originate in the underlying muscle. Here, arteries branch into smaller vessels, which then branch into the network of capillaries that permeate the dermis and subcutaneous tissue.

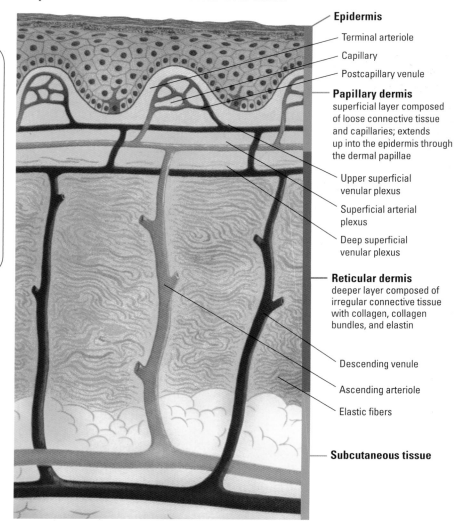

Only capillaries have walls thin enough to let solutes pass through. These thin walls allow nutrients and oxygen to pass from the bloodstream into the interstitial space around skin cells. At the same time, waste products pass into the capillaries and are carried away.

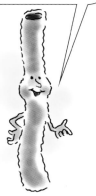

Epidermis

Terminal arteriole

Capillary

Postcapillary venule

Papillary dermis
superficial layer composed of loose connective tissue and capillaries; extends up into the epidermis through the dermal papillae

Upper superficial venular plexus

Superficial arterial plexus

Deep superficial venular plexus

Reticular dermis
deeper layer composed of irregular connective tissue with collagen, collagen bundles, and elastin

Descending venule

Ascending arteriole

Elastic fibers

Subcutaneous tissue

Physiology

Skin performs, or participates in, a host of vital functions and functions best when well hydrated. Well-hydrated skin supports ideal skin pH between 4.0 and 6.0. Alterations in skin pH increase susceptibility to infections. Damage to skin impairs its ability to carry out the many important functions of the skin.

Functions of the skin

Function		Description
	Protection	• Acts as a physical barrier to microorganisms and foreign matter • Protects the body against infection from the environment with the Langerhans cells (triggers immune system) • Protects underlying tissue and structures from mechanical injury • Prevents the loss of electrolytes, heat, water, proteins, and other substances to maintain homeostasis
	Sensory perception	• Contains nerve endings and sensory receptors (Merkel's cells) • Allows for perception of pain, pressure, heat, and cold to identify potential dangers and avoid injury
	Thermoregulation	• Contains nerves, blood vessels, and eccrine glands in the dermis to control body temperature • Causes blood vessels to constrict (reducing blood flow and conserving heat) when exposed to cold or internal body temperature falls • Causes small arteries in the skin to dilate and increases sweat production to promote cooling when skin becomes hot or internal body temperature rises
	Excretion	• Transmits trace amounts of water and body wastes to the environment • Allows the skin to maintain thermoregulation and electrolyte and hydration balances • Prevents dehydration by ensuring that the body doesn't lose too much water
	Metabolism	• Helps to maintain the mineralization of bones and teeth • Synthesizes vitamin D (which is crucial to the metabolism of calcium and phosphate) when exposed to the ultraviolet spectrum in sunlight
	Absorption	• Allows for the absorption of some drugs directly into the bloodstream

Aging and skin function

With aging, the skin undergoes a number of changes that increase the risk of wound development and impair the ability of wounds to heal. Skin changes begin at birth and continue throughout the lifespan. Aging skin loses firmness and elasticity related to changes in collagen and elastin production.

> As people age, their skin's ability to sense pressure, heat, and cold becomes impaired, even though the number of nerve endings in the skin remains unchanged.

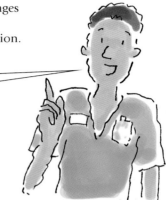

Youthful skin

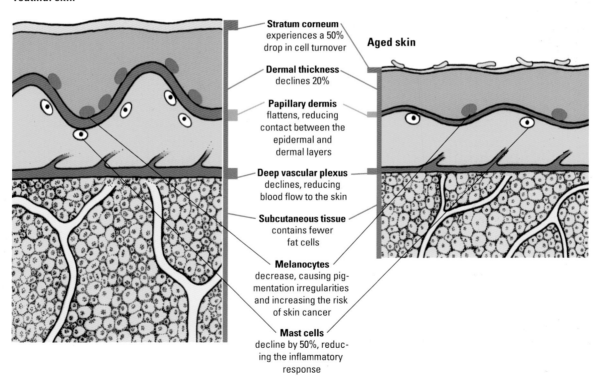

Aged skin

Stratum corneum experiences a 50% drop in cell turnover

Dermal thickness declines 20%

Papillary dermis flattens, reducing contact between the epidermal and dermal layers

Deep vascular plexus declines, reducing blood flow to the skin

Subcutaneous tissue contains fewer fat cells

Melanocytes decrease, causing pigmentation irregularities and increasing the risk of skin cancer

Mast cells decline by 50%, reducing the inflammatory response

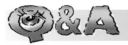

Able to label?

Identify the five layers of the epidermis indicated on this illustration.

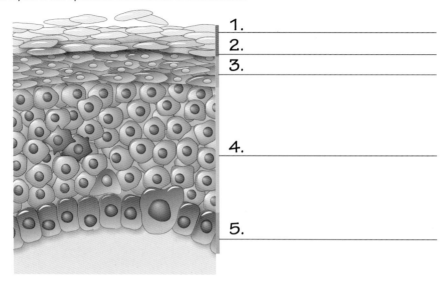

1. _____

2. _____

3. _____

4. _____

5. _____

Rebus riddle

Sound out each group of pictures and symbols to reveal an important fact about the skin.

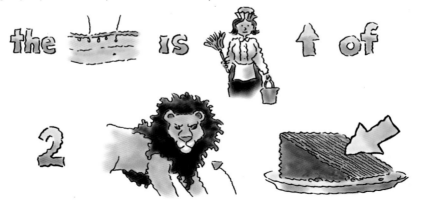

Selected References

Clark, R. A., & Kelly, A. P. (2016). Biology of wounds and wound care. *Taylor and Kelly's dermatology for skin of color 2/E*, 94. London: Elsevier.

Gilaberte, Y., Prieto-Torres, L., Pastushenko, I., & Juarranz, A. (2016). Anatomy and function of the skin. *Nanoscience in Dermatology*. New York: McGraw-Hill Medical Publishing Division.

Moissl-Eichinger, C., Probst, A. J., Birarda, G., Auerbach, A., Koskinen, K., Wolf, P., & Holman, H. Y. N. (2017). Human age and skin physiology shape diversity and abundance of Archaea on skin. *Scientific Reports, 7*.

Wong, R., Geyer, S., Weninger, W., Guimberteau, J. C., & Wong, J. K. (2016). The dynamic anatomy and patterning of skin. *Experimental Dermatology, 25*(2), 92–98.

Wound, Ostomy, Continence Nurses Society®, Doughty, D., & Moore, K. (2015). *Wound, Ostomy and Continence Nurses Society® core curriculum: Continence management*. Philadelphia, PA: Lippincott Williams & Wilkins.

Chapter 2

Wound healing

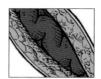

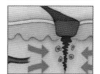

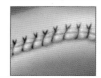

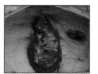

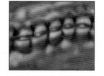

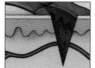

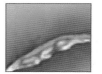

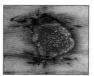

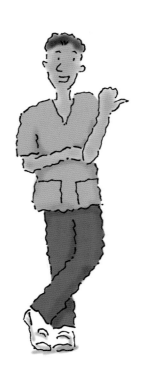

Types of wound healing

Any disruption in the skin and underlying structures is considered a wound. Humans typically heal along a "programmed" cascade when there is an acute injury. The extent and type of damage—as well as other intrinsic factors, such as patient circulation, nutrition, and hydration—influence the rate of wound repair. Wounds can heal, or close, through a series of phases. The closure of the wound also dictates how it will heal. There are 4 types of wound closures: primary, secondary, tertiary intention, and epithelization.

Primary intention

Wounds that heal through primary intention usually don't involve the loss of tissue. These wounds are closed with sutures or staples at the time of surgery, closing all layers of tissue. Examples include surgical wounds, superficial traumatic wounds, and first-degree sunburn.

Clean incision

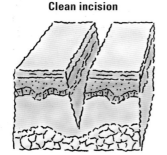

Wound has well-approximated edges.

Early suture

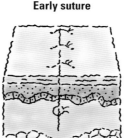

Clean edges can be pulled together neatly.

Hairline scar

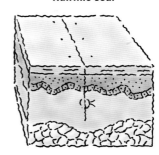

Because there's no loss of tissue and little risk of infection, these wounds usually heal in 4 to 14 days and result in minimal scarring.

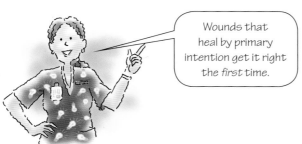

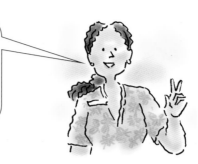

Wounds that heal by secondary intention need a second chance to get it right. Luckily, granulation tissue can "fill in" the gap.

Secondary intention

A wound that involves some degree of tissue loss heals by secondary intention. These full-thickness wounds fill in from the bottom with granulation tissue and then epithelize and scar. Pressure ulcers, burns, dehisced surgical wounds, and traumatic injuries are examples of this type of wound. These wounds take longer to heal, result in scarring, and have a higher rate of complications than do wounds that heal by primary intention.

Gaping irregular wound	**Granulation**	**Epithelium growth over scar**
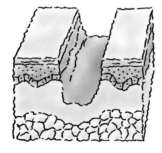	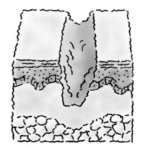	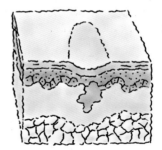
Edges can't be easily approximated.	Wound fills with granulation tissue.	A scar forms, and reepithelialization occurs, primarily from the wound edges.

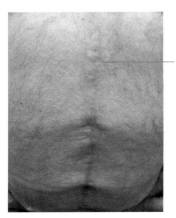

This wound was closed with primary intention, then there was wound dehiscence. Note the proximal end is a wider scar that healed by secondary intention.

Tertiary intention

Wounds are sometimes left open for several days to allow edema or infection to resolve or for exudate to drain. These wounds heal by tertiary intention, also known as *delayed primary closure*. After the problem resolves, these wounds are closed with sutures or some other type of skin closure.

Open wound

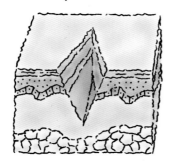

Wound is intentionally kept open (typically for 3 to 5 days) to allow edema or infection to resolve or to permit removal of exudate.

Increased granulation

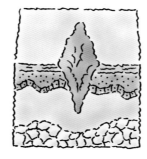

Wound fills with granulation tissue.

Late suturing with wide scar

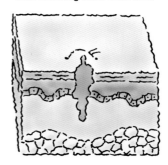

Wound is sutured late, and a wide scar results.

Wounds that heal by tertiary intention need three steps: draining, "filling" by granulation, and then suturing.

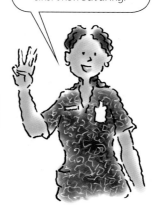

Epithelization

In this final process of wound healing, epithelial cells migrate across the wound bed. For partial-thickness wounds, those involving only the top layers of the skin (superficial dermis and epidermis), this is the primary method of healing. For example, with a knee abrasion, wound contracture and filling in with granulation tissue will not occur.

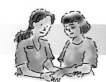

Special attention

Wound healing and bariatric patients

Bariatric patients are at risk for delayed wound healing due to:
• reduced tissue perfusion in adipose tissue and increased tension at the suture line caused by the weight of excess body fat
• excess skin folds (especially if the wound is within a fold or if a fold covers a suture line, which may keep the wound moist and allow bacteria to accumulate)
• associated medical conditions such as type 2 diabetes mellitus.

Bariatric patients are also at risk for dehiscence and evisceration because their diets may be seriously lacking in essential vitamins and minerals that are necessary for proper wound healing.

Phases of wound healing

The healing process is the same for all wounds, whether the cause is mechanical, chemical, or thermal. Health care professionals discuss the process of wound healing in four specific phases: hemostasis, inflammation, proliferation, and maturation (remodeling).

Wound healing process

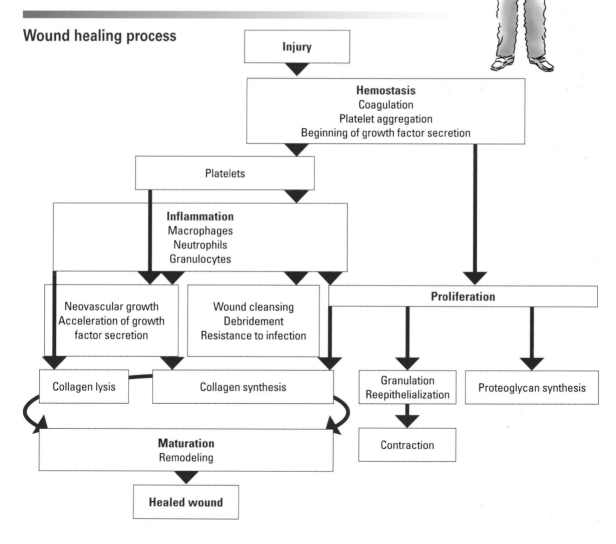

1 Hemostasis

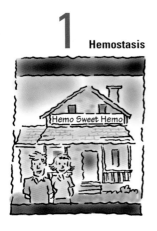

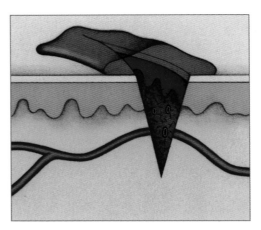

The injury causes an outflow of fluid, both blood and lymphatics, at the site. The body activates intrinsic and extrinsic factors to heal. When tissue is damaged, serotonin, histamine, prostaglandins, and blood from the injured vessels fill the area. Blood platelets form a clot, and fibrin in the clot binds the wound edges together. The inflammation stage is initiated during hemostasis, and this process may last a few days.

2 Inflammation

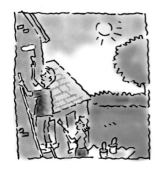

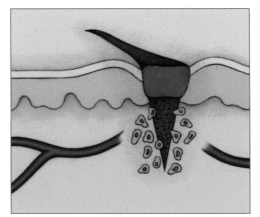

Lymphocytes initiate the inflammatory response, increasing capillary permeability. Wound edges swell. White blood cells from surrounding vessels move in and ingest bacteria and cellular debris, demolishing the clot and healing the wound. Redness, warmth, swelling, pain, and loss of function may occur. Platelets heavily secrete growth factors during this phase.

3 Proliferation

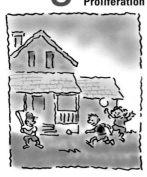

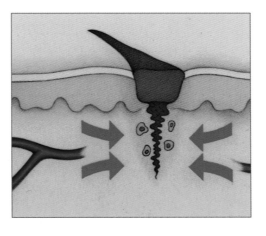

Adjacent healthy tissue supplies blood, nutrients, fibroblasts, proteins, and other building materials needed to form soft, pink, and highly vascular granulation tissue, which begins to fill and cover the area.

4 Maturation

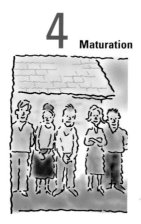

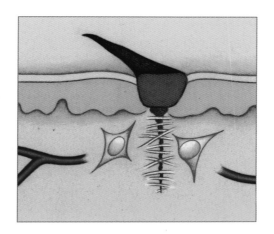

Fibroblasts in the granulation tissue secrete collagen, a gluelike substance. Collagen fibers crisscross the area, forming scar tissue. A new layer of surface cells replaces the layer that was destroyed. New, healthy tissue or granulation tissue appears.

Meanwhile, epithelial cells at the wound edge multiply and migrate toward the wound center. This epithelial tissue will be a light pink "halo" that grows around the edge of the wound until it fills the whole wound with a scar. As it heals, the color will be deposited into the wound that is the same color as the skin.

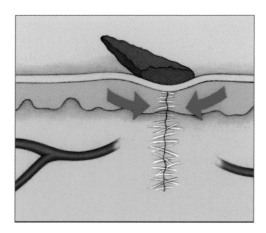

Over months or years, damaged tissue (including lymphatics, blood vessels, and stromal matrices) regenerates. Collagen fibers shorten, and the scar may diminish in size. Normal function may return, but the scar will only have approximately 80% of the strength of unwounded skin. Alternatively, the scar may hypertrophy, leading to the formation of a keloid and the development of contractures.

Wound healing: partial- versus full-thickness wounds

Partial-thickness wounds are wounds that involve the top layers of skin specifically the epidermal and dermal layers. Partial-thickness wounds heal by epithelization only.

Full-thickness wounds are wounds that extend through the dermis and into subdermal structures.

The more damage that is done to the tissues, the more the mechanisms of healing that are required. Full-thickness wounds will have scar evidence of healing.

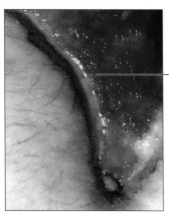

Full thickness wound with epithelial "halo". Epithelial tissue migrating from intact skin over granulation tissue.

Full-thickness wound around a colostomy.

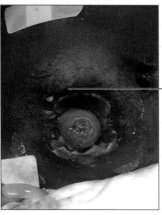

Note it is beginning to fill in with granulation tissue and has an epithelial halo starting.

Wound healing: acute versus chronic wounds

Simply put, acute wounds progress along the healing phases in an orderly predictable fashion. The mechanism of injury is easily identifiable in acute wounds, for example surgery or trauma. Delays in wound healing are typically minimal and easily addressed.

Chronic wounds are wounds that do not follow the healing process in an orderly, timely manner. Sometimes they "fall off" the healing cascade. Due to various factors, these wounds stall in one of the phases and require long-term follow-up.

Debridement may be used to convert a wound from a chronic to acute one. The debridement activates the healing cascade, and normal healing may commence. All systemic factors must be addressed, or the wound will not continue to heal along the cascade.

Recognizing wound failure to heal

Sign	Causes	Interventions
Wound bed		
Too dry	• Exposure of tissue and cells normally in a moist environment to air • Inadequate hydration	• Add moisture regularly. • Use a dressing that maintains moisture, such as a hydrocolloid or hydrogel dressing. • Reassess patient hydration status.
No change in size or depth for 2 weeks	• Pressure or trauma to the area • Poor nutrition, poor circulation, or inadequate hydration • Poor control of disease processes such as diabetes • Inadequate pain control • Infection	• Reassess the patient for local or systemic problems that impair wound healing, and intervene as necessary.
Increase in size or depth	• Debridement • Ischemia due to excess pressure or poor circulation • Infection	• Reassess the patient for local or systemic problems that impair wound healing, and intervene as necessary. • If caused by debridement, no intervention is necessary. • Poor circulation may not be resolvable, but consider adding warmth to the area and discussing with the qualified health care professional (QHP). • Administer a vasodilator or antiplatelet medication. • If caused by infection, apply topical antimicrobials or administer antibiotics, as ordered.
Necrosis	• Ischemia	• Consult the QHP regarding debridement if the remaining living tissue has adequate circulation.
Too wet and/or increase in drainage or change in drainage from clear to purulent	• Autolytic or enzymatic debridement • Increased bioburden from increasing colonization • Infection	• If caused by autolytic or enzymatic debridement, no intervention is necessary; an increase or change of color in drainage is expected because of the breakdown of dead tissue. Choose a dressing that adequately absorbs drainage. • If debridement isn't the cause, assess the wound for increased bioburden or for infection. • If caused by increased bioburden or infection, apply topical antimicrobials and/or administer antibiotics, as ordered.
Tunneling	• Pressure over bony prominences • Presence of foreign body • Deep infection	• Protect the area from pressure. • Irrigate and inspect the tunnel as carefully as possible for a hidden suture or leftover bit of dressing material. • If the tunnel doesn't shorten in length each week, thoroughly clean and obtain a tissue biopsy for infection and, with a chronic wound, for possible malignancy. • Address potential causes of shear if the wound is a pressure injury.

Recognizing wound failure to heal *(continued)*

Sign	Causes	Interventions
Wound edges		
Red, hot skin; tenderness; and induration	• Inflammation due to excess pressure or infection	• Protect the area from pressure. • If pressure relief doesn't resolve the inflammation within 24 hours, topical antimicrobial therapy may be indicated.
Maceration (white skin)	• Excess moisture	• Protect the skin with skin protective ointment, skin prep spray, or a barrier wipe. • If practical, consider a more absorptive dressing.
Rolled skin edges (epibole)	• Too-dry wound bed • Infection • Trauma • Overpacking	• Correct causal factor. • Consider moisture-retentive dressings, antimicrobial dressing. • If rolling isn't resolved in 1 week, debridement of the edges may be necessary.
Undermining or ecchymosis of surrounding skin (loose or bruised skin edges)	• Excess shearing force to the area	• Protect the area from shear, especially during patient transfers. • Address potential causes of shear. • Consider using a five-layer foam dressing.

Effects of aging on wound healing

Age itself is not a risk factor for failure to heal. Wound healing may not be defective, just delayed. Problems with delayed wound healing in a person with advanced age may be more a problem with other comorbidities that affect some older patients.

Factors that delay healing
- Slower turnover rate in epidermal cells
- Poor oxygenation of the wound (due to increasingly fragile capillaries and a reduction in skin vascularization or comorbidities such as pulmonary or cardiac issues)
- Impaired function of the respiratory or immune system
- Reduced dermal and subcutaneous mass (leading to an increased risk of chronic pressure ulcers/injuries)
- Lack of tensile strength in healed wounds, making them prone to reinjure

Factors that complicate healing
- Poor nutrition and hydration
- Presence of a chronic condition
- Use of multiple medications, including anti-inflammatory drugs and immuno-suppressants
- Decreased mobility
- Incontinence
- Extrinsic factors: smoking, radiation, chemotherapy, steroids

Physical changes from aging—such as a declining sense of smell and taste and decreased stomach motility—can affect a patient's nutritional and fluid intake.

Other factors can also affect our nutritional status, such as loose dentures, financial concerns, problems preparing or obtaining food, and mental status changes.

Complications of wound healing

Wound dehiscence
Dehiscence is a separation of skin and tissue layers. It's most likely to occur 3 to 11 days after the injury was sustained and may follow surgery.

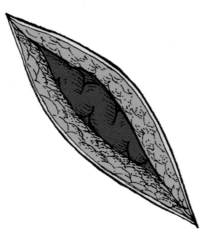

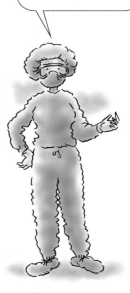

Dehiscence and evisceration may require emergency surgery, especially when an abdominal wound is involved. If a wound opens without evisceration, it may need to heal by secondary intention.

Evisceration of bowel loop
Evisceration is similar to dehiscence but involves protrusion of underlying visceral organs as well.

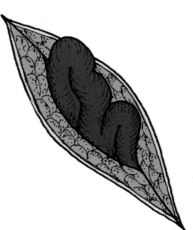

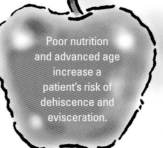

Poor nutrition and advanced age increase a patient's risk of dehiscence and evisceration.

Detecting wound dehiscence

Signs of dehiscence include an abscess or a gush of sanguineous fluid from the wound. The patient may also report a "popping" sensation at the wound site.

Dehisced abdominal wound (with a colostomy)

Healing dehisced abdominal wound by secondary intention

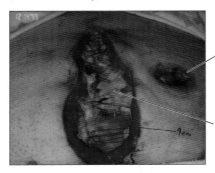

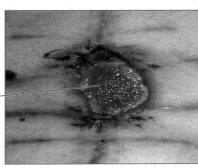

Colostomy

Red granulation tissue

Necrotic tissue

Take note

Documenting wound dehiscence and evisceration

5/24/18	0945	Wound Change: Wound 30 cm long approximated. Staples removed
		5/23/18. Dehiscence of distal 10 cm of midline abdominal incision.
		Periwound skin clean, dry intact. Scant amount of serosanguineous
		drainage on dressing. Superficial layers of tissue observed; no evis-
		ceration noted. Pt. placed in reclined position with knees flexed. Pt.
		states, "I felt something give when I coughed." Wound covered with
		sterile 4" x 4" gauze dampened with normal saline, edges protected
		with zinc paste, dry sterile dressing, tape to secure. P 100, BP 150/84,
		RR 18, T 98.6°F. Dr. McBride notified at 0930. Adhesive strips
		ordered and applied to wound. Pt. to be on bed rest until
		Dr. McBride visits at 1030. Pt. instructed to stay in bed with knees
		flexed and to call nurse for assistance with moving. Reviewed splint-
		ing incision with pillow during coughing or sneezing. Call bell placed
		within reach, and pt. demonstrated use. Pt. denies pain and is free
		from objective signs of discomfort. -----M.Fraser, RN

Infection

Infection is a relatively common complication of wound healing that should be addressed promptly.

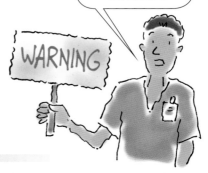

> Infection can lead to cellulitis or bacterial infection that spreads to surrounding tissue. So, be alert!

Signs of infection
- Redness and warmth of the margins and tissue around the wound
- Fever (temperature > 101.5°F)
- Edema
- Pain (or a sudden increase in pain)
- Purulent drainage
- Increase in exudate or a change in its color
- Odor
- Discoloration of granulation tissue
- Further wound breakdown or lack of progress toward healing

Recognizing wound infection

Clean wound

The wound here is healing properly. It's clean and has no redness, swelling, or drainage.

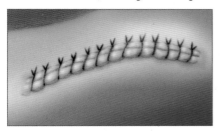

Infected wounds

These wounds show signs of infection.

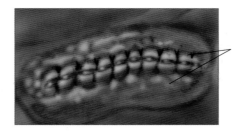

Redness and swelling along the incision line and in surrounding tissue

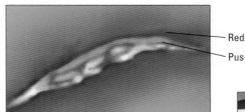

Redness

Pus

Dotted area outlines erythema for this infected wound. Compare to non-infected wound.

Fistulas and sinus tracts

A fistula is an abnormal passage between an organ or a vessel and another organ, vessel, or area of the skin. A sinus tract, also known as *tunneling*, is a channel that extends through part of a wound and into adjacent tissue. These complications can result in dead space and infection.

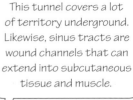

This tunnel covers a lot of territory underground. Likewise, sinus tracts are wound channels that can extend into subcutaneous tissue and muscle.

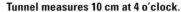

Tunnel measures 10 cm at 4 o'clock.

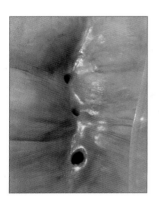

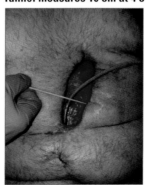

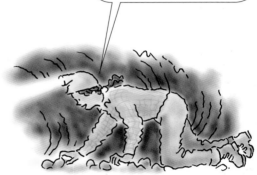

Undermining

Undermining is tissue destruction that occurs around a wound's edges, causing the skin to come away from the base of the wound (even though it may appear intact). This injury may be the result of friction and shear. It can develop into sinus tracts to nearby tissue.

Undermining should be carefully probed to determine how far it extends under intact skin.

Undermining is tissue destruction around the borders of a wound. It results in a wound bed that extends under the skin.

This wound demonstrates 2 cm undermining from 7 to 9 o'clock.

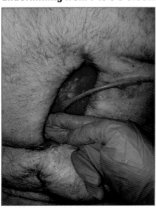

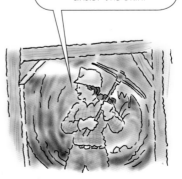

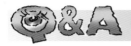

Matchmaker

Match each illustration to the proper phase of wound healing.

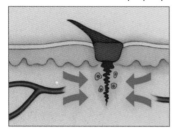

A.

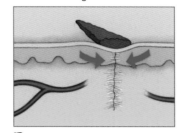

B.

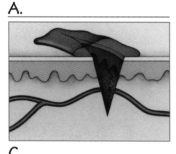

C.

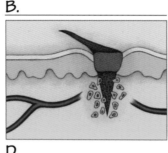

D.

1. Hemostasis

2. Inflammation

3. Proliferation

4. Maturation

My word!

Unscramble the names of four complications of wound healing. Then use the circled letters to answer the question posed.

Question: Which sign of failure to heal is caused by ischemia and requires wound debridement?

1. icravesitone __ __ ◯ __ __ __ ◯ __ __ __ __ __

2. sciencehed __ ◯ __ __ ◯ __ __ ◯ __ __

3. niceifnot __ __ __ __ ◯ __ __ ◯ __

4. usaflit __ __ ◯ __ __ __ __

Answer: __ __ __ __ __ __ __

Selected References

Doughty, D., & McNichol, L. (2016). *WOCN core curriculum wound management.* Philadelphia, PA: Wolters Kluwer.

Mercandetti, M., et al. (2017). Wound healing and repair. *Medscape.* Accessed September 26, 2017 at http://emedicine.medscspe.com/article/1298129-overview

Pastar, I., Stojadinovic, O., Yin, N. C., Ramirez, H., Nusbaum, A. G., Sawaya, A., … Tomic-Canic, M. (2014). Epithelization in wound healing: A comprehensive review. *Advances in Wound Care, 3*(7), 445–464.

Chapter 3

Wound assessment

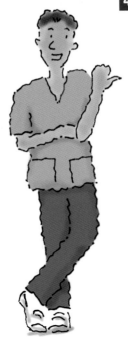

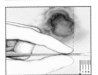

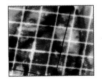
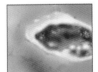
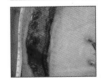

Wound classification

The words used to describe a wound must communicate the same thing to members of the health care team, insurance companies, regulators, the patient's family, and, ultimately, the patient himself. The best way to classify wounds is to use the basic system described here, which focuses on three categories of fundamental characteristics:

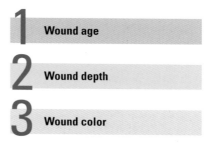

1 Wound age

2 Wound depth

3 Wound color

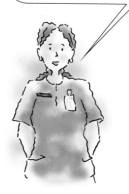

Even when the wound bed appears healthy, red, and moist, if healing fails to progress, consider the wound to be chronic.

Wound age

The first step in classifying a wound is to determine whether the wound is acute or chronic. Be careful; you can't base your determination solely on time because no set time frame specifies when an acute wound becomes chronic.

Characteristics of acute and chronic wounds

Acute
- New or relatively new wound
- Occurs suddenly
- Healing progresses in a timely, orderly, and predictable manner
- Typically heals by primary intention
- Examples: Surgical and traumatic wounds

Chronic
- May develop over time
- Healing has slowed or stopped
- Typically heals by secondary intention
- Examples: Pressure, vascular, and diabetic ulcers

Wound depth

Wound depth can be classified as partial thickness or full thickness.

> In the case of pressure injuries/ulcers, wound depth allows you to stage the injury/ulcer according to the classification system developed by the National Pressure Ulcer Advisory Panel. (See Chapter 6, Pressure ulcers.)

Partial-thickness wound

Partial-thickness wounds involve only the epidermis or extend into the dermis but not through it.

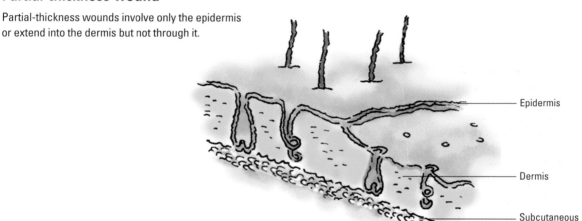

Epidermis

Dermis

Subcutaneous tissue

Full-thickness wound

Full-thickness wounds extend through the dermis into tissues beneath and may expose adipose tissue, muscle, or bone.

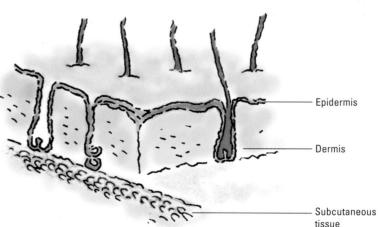

Epidermis

Dermis

Subcutaneous tissue

Measuring wound depth

To measure the depth of a wound, you'll need gloves, a cotton-tipped swab, and a disposable measuring device. This method can also be used to measure wound tunneling or undermining.

1 Put on gloves and gently insert the swab into the deepest portion of the wound.

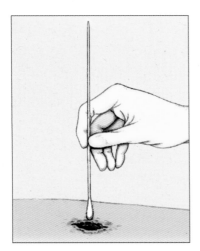

2 Grasp the swab with your fingers at the point that corresponds to the wound's margin. You can carefully mark the swab where it meets the edge of the skin.

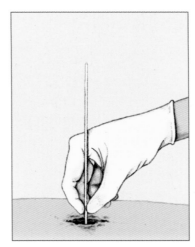

3 Remove the swab and measure the distance from your fingers or from the mark on the swab to the end of the swab to determine the depth.

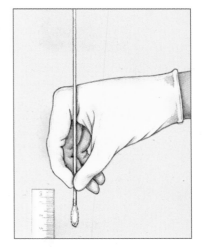

Wound color

The Red-Yellow-Black Classification System is a commonly used approach that can help you determine how well a wound is healing and develop effective wound care management plans.

Red wounds

Red indicates normal healing. When a wound begins to heal, a layer of granulation tissue covers the wound bed. Granulation tissue is shiny and bright with a bumpy surface.

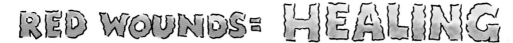

Granulation tissue in an abdominal wound

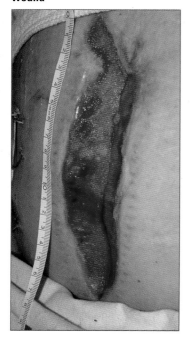

Yellow wounds

Fibrin leftover from the healing process usually appears as avascular yellow slough or dead tissue on the wound base. This slough, or soft necrotic tissue, provides a medium for bacterial growth.

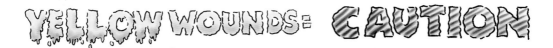

Sacral pressure injury/ulcer with 75% of the surface area covered in yellow necrotic slough

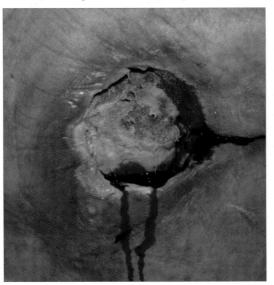

Diabetic foot ulcer with a slough-covered base and calloused edges.

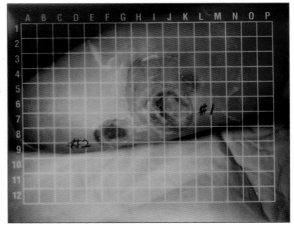

Black wounds

Black, the least healthy wound color, signals necrosis. Avascular dead tissue (known as *eschar*) slows healing and provides a site for microorganisms to proliferate.

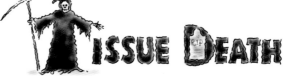

Black pressure ulcer

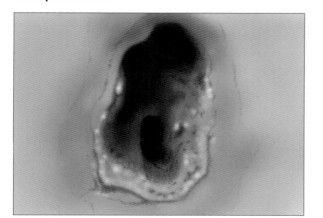

Black ischemic toe ulcers

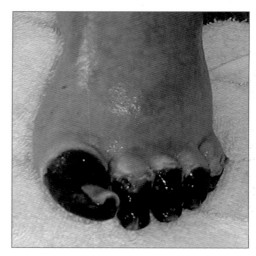

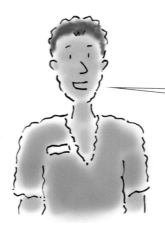

When eschar covers a wound, accurate assessment of wound depth is difficult and should be deferred until eschar is removed.

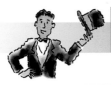

Best dressed

Tailoring wound care to wound color

Wound color	Management technique—Base selection of dressing choice on the amount of exudate in the wound bed.
Red	• Cover the wound, keep it moist and clean, and protect it from trauma. • Use a transparent film, hydrogel, foam, fiber, or hydrocolloid dressing (depending on amount of wound exudate) to insulate and protect the wound.
Yellow	• Clean the wound and remove the yellow layer. • Cover the wound with a moisture-retentive dressing (such as a transparent film, hydrocolloid, hydrogel, or foam dressing or a moist gauze dressing with or without a debriding enzyme). See Chapter 11 for more on dressings. • Consider pulsatile lavage or ultrasonic debridement.
Black	• Debride the wound as ordered. Use a selective debridement enzyme product (such as collagenase), conservative sharp debridement, or pulsatile lavage. • For wounds with inadequate blood supply and uninfected heel ulcers, don't debride. Keep them clean and dry.

Classifying multicolored wounds

If you note two or even all three colors in a wound, classify the wound according to the least healthy color present. For example, if your patient's wound appears both red and yellow, classify it as a yellow wound.

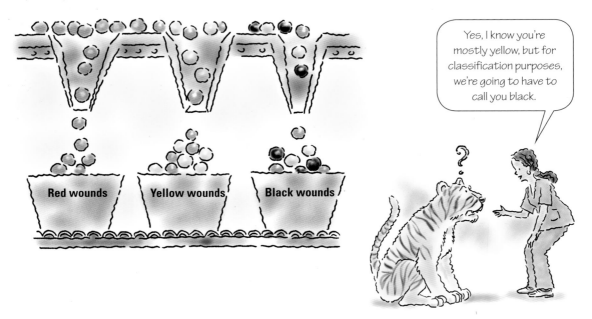

Red wounds   Yellow wounds   Black wounds

Yes, I know you're mostly yellow, but for classification purposes, we're going to have to call you black.

Wound terminology

Every wound has a different size, shape, and color, which can make accurate documentation challenging. However, understanding and using standard terminology can make the job easier.

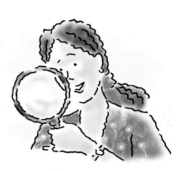

Call 'em like you see 'em

When you visually examine a wound, look for the following key characteristics.

What do you see?

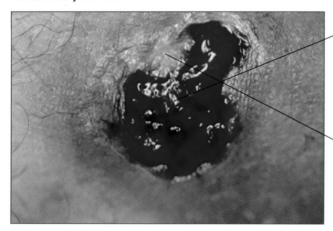

Red, bumpy, shiny tissue in the base of an ulcer
* This indicates **granulation tissue**.
* As a wound heals, it develops more and more granulation tissue.

  Beware, beefy red tissue that is friable (bleeds easily) may indicate excessive bioburden in the wound. This colonized wound needs to be treated topically.

Pale or pearly pink skin
* This indicates **epithelial tissue**.
* Epithelial tissue first appears at ulcer borders in full-thickness wounds and as islands around hair follicles in partial-thickness wounds.

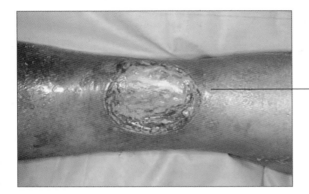

Moist yellow, tan, or gray area of tissue that's separating from viable tissue
- This is **slough** and indicates soft, necrotic tissue.
- Slough provides an ideal medium for bacterial growth.

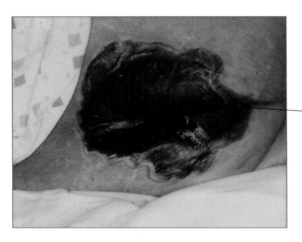

Thick, hard, leathery black tissue
- This is **eschar** and indicates dry, necrotic tissue.
- For healing to occur, necrotic tissue, drainage, and metabolic wastes must be removed.

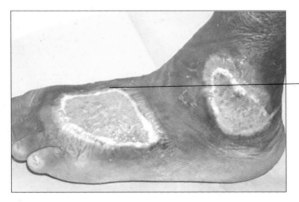

Waterlogged skin; possibly white at the wound edges
- This indicates **macerated tissue**.
- A dressing that provides too much moisture or that is not absorptive enough can cause maceration of surrounding skin, unless the skin is protected.
- Other common causes of maceration include wound drainage or contamination with urine or feces.

Wound drainage

A thorough wound assessment includes assessing drainage. To begin collecting information about wound drainage, inspect the dressing as it's removed and record your findings.

Drainage descriptors

Description	Color and consistency
Serous	• Clear or light yellow • Thin and watery
Sanguineous	• Red (with fresh blood) • Thin
Serosanguineous	• Pink to light red • Thin • Watery
Purulent	• Creamy yellow, green, white, or tan • Thick and opaque

Take note

Documenting wound drainage

03/30/18	1330	Dressing on abdominal surgical
		site changed. Pt. medicated with
		2 mg of morphine sulfate at
		1315 for comfort. Dressing was
		dry and intact. No oozing from
		edges of dressing noted at this
		time. Dressing removed using
		adhesive remover. Moderate
		amount of serosanguineous
		drainage present on interior of
		dressing. No odor from drainage
		noted. Patient tolerated proce-
		dure without complaint of pain.
		___ *Bob White, R.N*

Wound measurement

When measuring a wound, you must determine its length, width, and depth. (Measuring wound depth is described on page 32.) You must also measure the surrounding areas.

1 Length

• Measure the greatest length with a head-to-toe orientation using a centimeter ruler.
• In this photo, note the line used to illustrate length.

2 Width

• Next, determine the longest distance across the wound (side to side), at a 90-degree angle to the length.
• In this photo, note the relationship between length and width.

3 Surrounding areas

• Note areas of erythematous (reddened), intact skin; indurated (or hard) skin; and white (macerated) skin.
• These areas are measured and recorded as surrounding erythema, induration, and maceration, not as part of the wound itself.

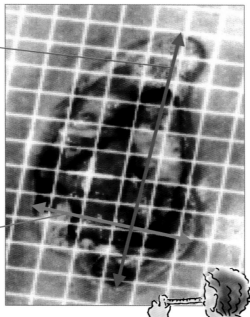

Measuring wound undermining and tunneling

Undermining, tunneling, and sinus tracts were discussed in Chapter 2. Because tunneling and undermining may be more extensive in one part of a wound than another, measuring and documenting the location (use a clock face) is important.

Probing the issue

• Put on clean or sterile gloves based on your facility policy. Gently probe the wound bed and edges with a sterile applicator to assess for wound undermining or tunneling.
• Gently insert the applicator around the wound edges for undermining or into the wound in the direction where the deepest tunneling occurs. Below is a photo of undermining measurement.

Marking progress

• Grasp the applicator where it meets the wound edge.
• Remove the applicator, keeping your hand in place, and place it next to the measuring guide to determine the measurement of the undermining in centimeters, as shown below.

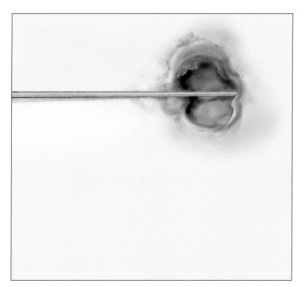

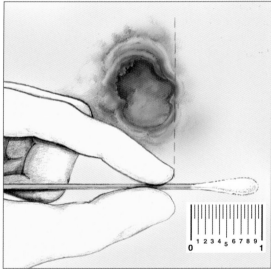

Wound documentation

Proper documentation accurately portrays the characteristics of a wound and its status in the healing process.

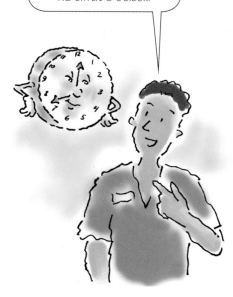

You can use the face of a clock to help document the direction of undermining and tunneling. For example, "Tunnel is 1.3 cm at 8 o'clock."

memory board

Use the mnemonic device **WOUNDD PICTURE** to help you recall and organize all of the key facts that should be included in your documentation of a wound:

Wound or ulcer location

Odor (in room or just when wound is uncovered)

Ulcer category, stage (for pressure injuries/ulcers) or classification (for diabetic ulcer), and depth (partial thickness or full thickness)

Necrotic tissue

Dimension (shape, length, width, and depth)

Drainage color, consistency, and amount (scant, moderate, or large)

Pain (when it occurs, what relieves it, patient's description, and patient's rating on scale of 0 to 10)

Induration (hard or soft surrounding tissue)

Color of wound bed (red, yellow, black, or combination)

Tunneling (length and direction—toward the patient's right, left, head, or feet)

Undermining (record length and direction, using clock references to describe)

Redness or other discoloration in surrounding skin

Edge of skin loose or tightly adhered and flat or rolled under

What's missing from this picture?

Wound photography may be a routine part of your facility's wound documentation system. Photographs can provide benchmarks for and facilitate documentation of wound healing.

Even though a picture may be "worth a thousand words," remember that your assessment skills and personal observations are still essential because many wound characteristics can't be recorded accurately—or at all—on film. For example, look at the photograph below and consider which wound characteristics you can't assess. Examples include:

* location
* depth
* tunnel measurement
* odor
* feel of surrounding tissue
* pain.

All wound assessment information is needed if the health care team is to make sound treatment decisions.

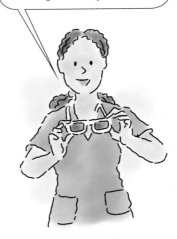

A special technology called *sterophotogrammetry* involves using overlapping photographs to provide a three-dimensional wound image. I guess I won't be needing these anymore then.

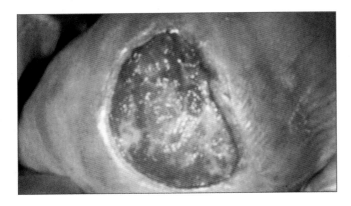

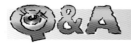

Matchmaker

Match each photo with the terminology that describes the characteristics of the wound.

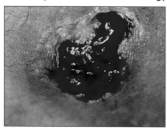

1. _____

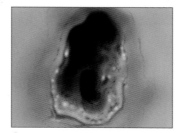

2. _____

A. Macerated tissue

B. Granulation tissue

C. Eschar

D. Slough

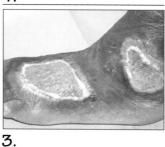

3. _____

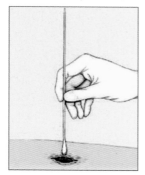

4. _____

Show and tell

Describe the three steps used to measure wound depth that are shown here.

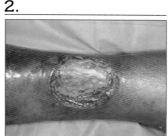

1. _____
_____
_____

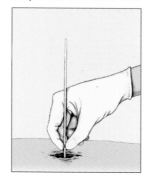

2. _____
_____
_____

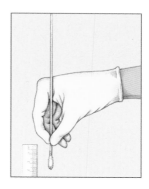

3. _____
_____
_____

Selected References

Baranoski, S., & Ayello, E. A. (2016). *Wound care essentials* (4th ed.). Philadelphia, PA: Lippincott Williams & Wilkins.

Doughty, D., & McNichol, L. (Eds.) (2016). *Wound Ostomy and Continence Nurses Society core curriculum: Wound management*. Philadelphia, PA: Wolters Kluwer.

Chapter 4

Wound care procedures

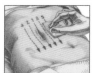
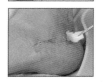
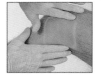
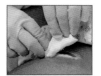
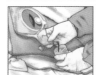
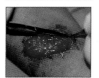
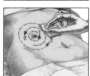
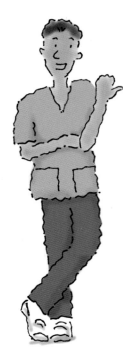

Cleaning a wound

The goal of wound cleaning is to remove debris and contaminants from the wound without damaging healthy tissue. After an initial cleaning, wounds should be cleaned before a new dressing is applied and as needed.

Step by step

As you follow these steps, be sure to observe standard precautions. Follow facility protocols regarding use of clean or sterile technique.

1 **Remove the soiled dressing.**
Put on clean gloves. Roll or lift an edge of the dressing, and then gently remove it while support-ing the surrounding skin. When possible, remove the dressing in the direction of hair growth.

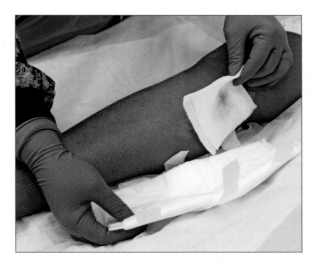

2 **Inspect the dressing and wound.**
Note the color, amount, and odor of drainage and necrotic debris.

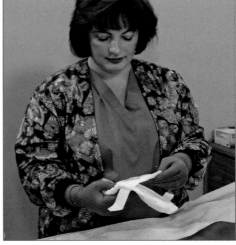

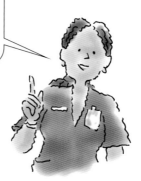

When cleaning a wound, move from the least contaminated area to the most contaminated area. Also, be sure to use a clean gauze pad for each wipe.

Cleaning techniques

To clean a linear-shaped wound (such as an incision), gently wipe from top to bottom in one motion, starting directly over the wound and moving outward, as shown below.

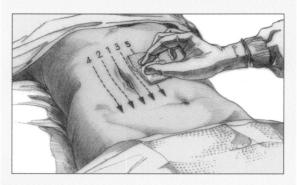

3 **Clean the wound.**
Moisten gauze pads either by dipping the pads in wound cleaning solution and wringing out excess or by using a spray bottle to apply solution to the gauze.

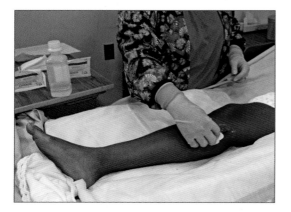

For an open wound (such as a pressure injury/ulcer), gently wipe in concentric circles, starting directly over the wound and moving outward, as shown below.

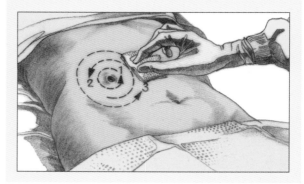

4 **Dry the wound.**
Using the same procedure as for cleaning a wound, dry the wound using dry gauze pads; pat dry; do not rub.

5 **Reassess the condition of the skin and wound.**
Note the character of the clean wound bed and surrounding skin.

Wound reassessment algorithm

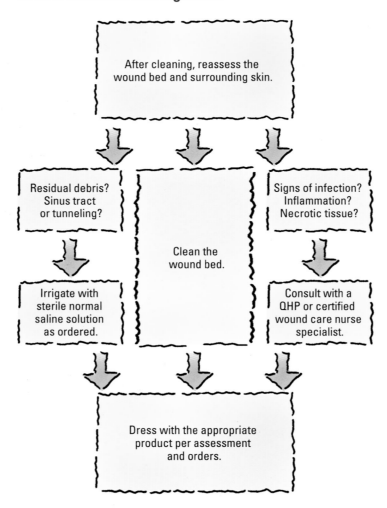

6 Remove soiled gloves, and replace. Dress the wound, filling dead space if indicated, as ordered.

Choosing a cleaning agent

The type of cleaning agent you'll use on a wound depends on the wound type and characteristics.

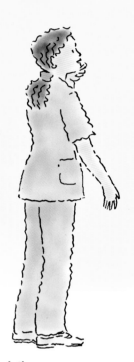

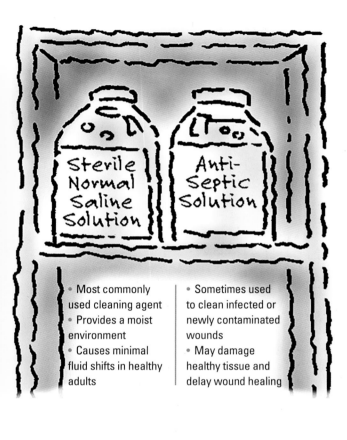

- Most commonly used cleaning agent
- Provides a moist environment
- Causes minimal fluid shifts in healthy adults

- Sometimes used to clean infected or newly contaminated wounds
- May damage healthy tissue and delay wound healing

Types of antiseptic solutions

Acetic acid	Sodium hypochlorite (Dakin's solution)	Povidone-iodine	Chlorhexidine
• Used to treat *Pseudomonas* infection • Verify active infection by culture before use • 0.5% to 5% strength depending on order	• Used to kill Gram-negative bacteria per culture • Slightly dissolves necrotic tissue • Must be freshly prepared every 48 hours and away from sunlight	• Used to kill broad spectrum of bacteria • May dry and stain the surrounding skin; protect from contact • Toxic with pro-longed use or over large areas • Avoid use in patients with thyroid disease	• Used to kill Gram-positive and Gram-negative bacteria • Must be diluted • Do not use on face, or mucous membranes

Watch for patient sensitivity to povidone-iodine.

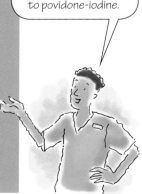

Irrigating a wound

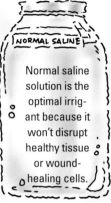

Normal saline solution is the optimal irrigant because it won't disrupt healthy tissue or wound-healing cells.

Step by step

As you follow these steps, be sure to observe standard precautions and maintain clean or sterile technique per your facility policy.

Irrigation serves to:
- clean tissues
- flush cell debris and drainage from an open wound
- prevent premature surface healing over an abscess pocket or infected tract.

1 **Prepare the solution and equipment.**
Fill the irrigating device with irrigating solution.

2 **Irrigate the entire wound thoroughly.**
Use a face shield, or mask and goggles, in case of a splash. Gently instill a slow, steady stream of solution into the wound (below left). Make sure the solution flows from the clean area to the dirty area of the wound to prevent contamination of clean tissue. To prevent tissue damage, don't force the needle or angiocatheter into the wound. Irrigate until you've administered the prescribed amount of solution or until the solution returns clear. Note the amount of solution administered. Keep the patient positioned to allow complete wound drainage (below right).

Devices used to irrigate a wound should provide gentle, low-pressure irrigation and may include a bulb syringe or a 35-ml piston syringe with an 18-gauge needle or angiocatheter.

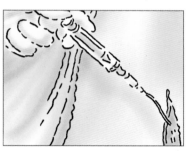

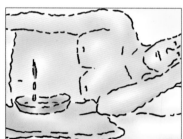

3 **Clean and dry the skin.**
Use normal saline solution on the periwound skin, and then pat it dry with gauze.

4 **Dress the wound (and fill the dead space if indicated) as ordered.**

Filling dead space

Filling dead space in a wound prevents surface healing before deep healing. The type of material used depends on the size of the wound and the amount of exudate. If using gauze, consider using roll gauze as you will not leave a piece behind on removal!

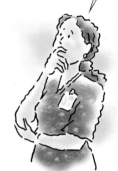

Times have changed! Cotton mesh gauze used to be the standard. Today, you have more options.

Step by step

As you follow these steps, be sure to observe standard precautions.

1 **Make sure the material is moist.**
Use a slight amount of sterile normal saline solution if needed (draining wounds do not usually need added moisture).

2 **Fill the dead space.**
Use sterile forceps and cotton-tipped applicators as needed.
—Fluff the moist sterile pad or strip to unclump it.
—Loosely but thoroughly fill the dead space in the wound. Note that "packing" the wound too tightly can create pressure damage on the granulating cells.
—Cover all the wound surfaces and edges.
—Keep dressing in the wound bed because moist dressings can macerate intact tissue.

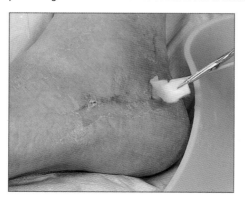
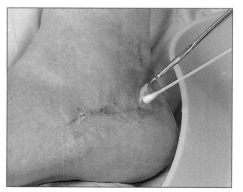

3 **Dress with dry sterile gauze.**

Dressing a wound

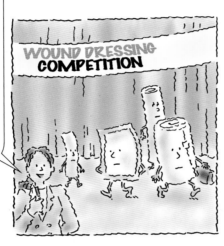

I'm here at the annual Wound Dressing Competition. As any fan of this competition knows, the winning dressing always provides an optimal environment in which the body can heal.

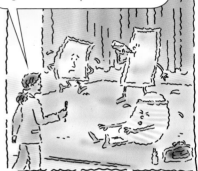

Competition is fierce. Contestants are judged on their ability to keep wounds moist, absorb drainage, conform to the wound, and be comfortable. Let's go to the competition floor.

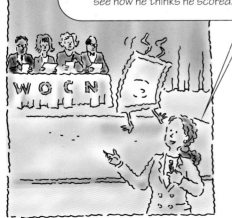

The composite dressing is taking his turn. He has scored a perfect 10 in his compulsories and is now performing his individual program. What a unique combination! Let's see how he thinks he scored.

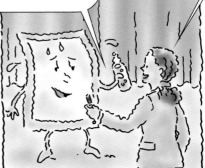

I did my best in adhering to the surrounding skin, decreasing the need for a secondary dressing, and showing my user-friendly side. Let's hope the judges also find me cost-effective.

Can I tell it like it is? I think you've impressed the judges. We'll have to see how the other contestants perform, though.

Wound dressing algorithm

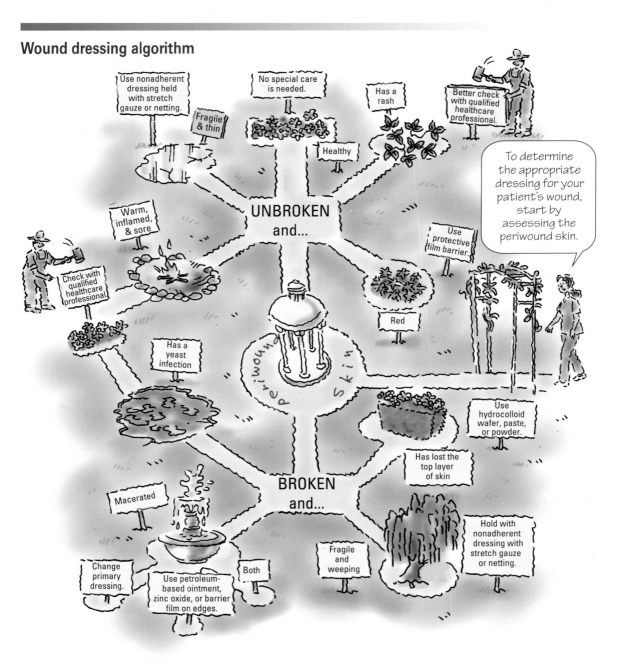

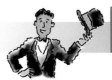

Best dressed

Step-by-step wound dressing

Regardless of the dressing or topical agent you use, follow your facility's protocol or the manufacturer's instructions for applying the wound dressing.

Type of dressing	Application method
Alginate	• Apply the dressing to the wound surface. • Cover the area with a secondary dressing (such as gauze pads, ABDs, or transparent film), as ordered. • Secure the dressing with tape or elastic netting. • If the wound is heavily draining, change the dressing once or twice daily for the first 3 to 5 days. As drainage decreases, change the dressing less frequently—every 2 to 4 days or as ordered. When the drainage stops or the wound bed looks dry, stop using alginate dressings.
Foam	• Gently lay the dressing over the wound. • Use tape, elastic netting, or gauze to hold the dressing in place if the foam does not have an adhesive border. • Change the dressing when the foam no longer absorbs exudate.
Hydrocolloid	• Choose a clean, dry, presized dressing or cut one to overlap the wound by about 1″ (2.5 cm). • Remove the dressing from its package. • Pull the release paper from the adherent side of the dressing. • Apply the dressing to the wound, carefully smoothing out wrinkles and avoiding stretching the dressing. • Hold the dressing in place with your hand (the warmth from your hand will mold the dressing to the skin). • If the dressing's edges need to be secured with tape, apply a skin sealant to the intact skin around the wound. After the area dries, tape the dressing to the skin. The sealant protects the skin from tape burns and skin stripping and promotes tape adherence. Avoid using tension or pressure when you apply the tape. • Change the dressing every 3 to 7 days as necessary; change it immediately if the patient complains of pain, the dressing no longer adheres, or leakage occurs.

Type of dressing	Application method
Hydrogel	• Apply a moderate amount of gel to the wound bed, enough to cover the surface. • Cover the area with a secondary dressing (nonadherent gauze, or transparent film). • Change the dressing daily or as needed to keep the wound bed moist. • If the dressing you select comes in sheet form, cut the dressing to overlap the wound by 1″ (2.5 cm), protect periwound skin with a barrier; then apply as you would a hydrocolloid dressing. *Note:* Hydrogel dressings also come as prepackaged, saturated gauze and gauze strips for wounds with cavities that require "dead space" to be filled. Follow the manufacturer's directions to apply these dressings. 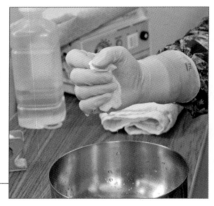
Moist saline gauze	• Moisten the dressing with normal saline solution. • Wring out excess fluid. • Open gauze pads and "fluff" gauze. • Gently place the "fluffed" dressing into the wound, molding the moist gauze around the wound. • To separate surfaces within the wound, gently guide the gauze between opposing wound surfaces. To avoid damage to tissues, don't overfill with the gauze. • Apply a sealant or barrier to protect the surrounding skin from moisture. • Change the dressing frequently enough to keep the wound moist, at least every 12 hours or three times per day. 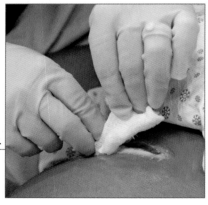
Transparent	• Select a dressing to overlap the wound by 1″ to 2″ (2.5 to 5 cm). • Apply a sealant or barrier to protect the surrounding skin from moisture. • Gently lay the dressing over the wound; avoid wrinkling the dressing. To prevent shearing force, don't stretch the dressing over the wound. Press firmly on the edges of the dressing to promote adherence. • Change the dressing every 3 to 5 days, depending on the amount of drainage. If the seal is no longer secure, change the dressing.

Applying a wound pouch

A wound with copious drainage may need to have a pouch applied. A wound pouch collects drainage and helps protect the surrounding skin.

Step by step

When applying a wound pouch, wear a gown and a face shield or mask and goggles in case the drainage splashes. Be sure to follow standard precautions when performing the following steps.

1 **Measure the wound.**
Use a disposable measuring tape to obtain the wound's length and width.

3 **Apply a skin protectant as needed.**
Note that some protectants are incorporated within the wafer and also provide adhesion.

2 **Cut an opening in the wafer.**
The opening should be 3/8″ (1 cm) larger than the wound (as shown below).

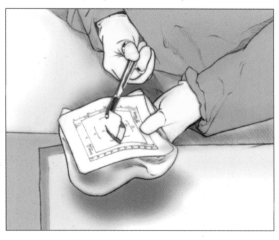

4 **Press the contoured pouch opening around the wound.**
Start at the lowest edge of the wound to catch any drainage (as shown below). (Note that this pouch was placed horizontally on the patient to facilitate emptying.)
−Make sure that the drainage port at the bottom of the pouch is closed firmly to prevent leaks.
−Be gentle but firm to avoid causing pain; offer to hold the wafer in place while the patient presses, if preferred.

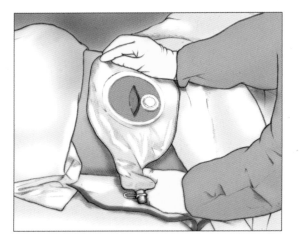

5 **Empty the pouch when 1/3 full.**
Empty the pouch into a graduated biohazard container (as shown below).
−Note the color, consistency, odor, and amount of fluid.

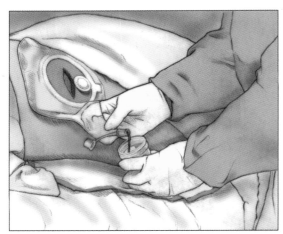

6 **Change the pouch as needed.**
Only change the pouch if it leaks or fails to adhere as more frequent changes may irritate the patient's skin.

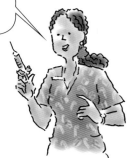

The surface swab technique obtains bacteria colonized only on the wound's surface. For a more accurate culture, needle aspiration of fluid or punch tissue biopsy should be used.

Collecting a wound culture

Heavily colonized and infected wounds (those with heavy bacterial or fungal overgrowth) are unable to properly heal. Cultures can help to determine the involved organism and guide treatment. One common wound culture collection method is the surface swab technique. Other methods, including syringe aspiration and punch tissue biopsy, are performed by qualified health care professionals.

Step by step

When obtaining a wound culture, follow standard precautions and maintain sterile technique throughout each of these steps.

1

Inspect and irrigate.
- Cleanse wound w/ NSS
- Remove/debride nonviable tissue and blot with sterile gauze
- Wait 2 to 5 minutes.

2

Swab
- Identify a healthy area of wound about 1 cm² (*Do not culture exudate, pus, eschar, or heavily fibrous tissue*)
- Moisten the swab with nonpreserved NSS if the ulcer bed is dry
- Rotate the end of a sterile applicator over a 1-cm² area for 5 seconds (technique suggests alginate tipped applicator). Apply sufficient pressure to swab to cause tissue fluid to be expressed.

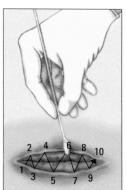
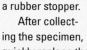

3

Place the swab in the appropriate culture medium
- When tip of swab is saturated, break tip using sterile technique into a collection device designed for quantitative cultures
- If the wound is open and has viable tissue, immediately place the swab in an aerobic culture tube. If the wound has necrotic tissue or sinus tracts, obtain both an aerobic and an anaerobic culture.

4

Label the culture tube.
Follow the facility policy. Include the patient's name, the date and time, the source location of the specimen, and your name or initials. You may be asked about any antibiotics the patient is taking. Immediately send the tube to the laboratory.

Collecting an anaerobic specimen
Because most anaerobes die when exposed to oxygen, they must be transported in tubes filled with carbon dioxide or nitrogen. Before specimen collection, the small inner tube containing the swab is held in place with a rubber stopper.
After collecting the specimen, quickly replace the swab in the inner tube and depress the plunger to separate the inner tube from the stopper. The swab is forced into the larger tube, exposing the specimen to a carbon dioxide–rich environment.

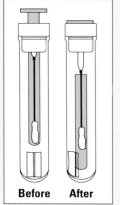

Before   **After**

Debriding a wound

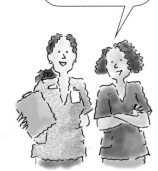

There's more than one way to debride a wound.

Debridement is the removal of necrotic (dead) tissue and debris (such as eschar and slough) from a wound. When combined with optimal nutrition, circulation, mobility, and attitude toward healing, debridement can help to promote wound healing.

Understanding debridement methods

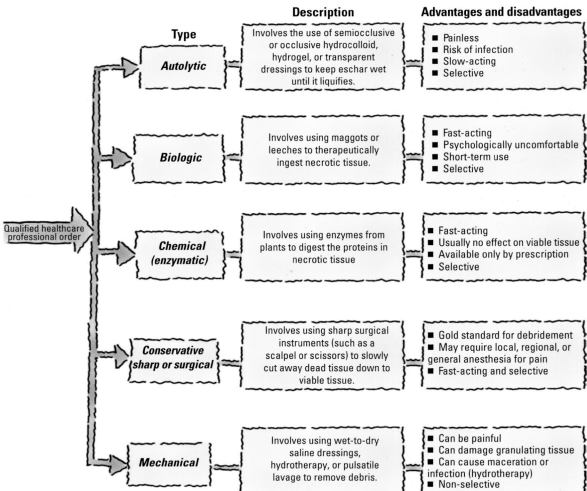

	Type	Description	Advantages and disadvantages
Qualified healthcare professional order	**Autolytic**	Involves the use of semiocclusive or occlusive hydrocolloid, hydrogel, or transparent dressings to keep eschar wet until it liquifies.	■ Painless ■ Risk of infection ■ Slow-acting ■ Selective
	Biologic	Involves using maggots or leeches to therapeutically ingest necrotic tissue.	■ Fast-acting ■ Psychologically uncomfortable ■ Short-term use ■ Selective
	Chemical (enzymatic)	Involves using enzymes from plants to digest the proteins in necrotic tissue	■ Fast-acting ■ Usually no effect on viable tissue ■ Available only by prescription ■ Selective
	Conservative sharp or surgical	Involves using sharp surgical instruments (such as a scalpel or scissors) to slowly cut away dead tissue down to viable tissue.	■ Gold standard for debridement ■ May require local, regional, or general anesthesia for pain ■ Fast-acting and selective
	Mechanical	Involves using wet-to-dry saline dressings, hydrotherapy, or pulsatile lavage to remove debris.	■ Can be painful ■ Can damage granulating tissue ■ Can cause maceration or infection (hydrotherapy) ■ Non-selective

Assisting in sharp debridement

Nonviable tissue

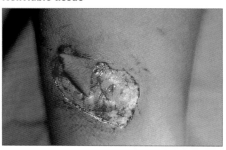

Conservative sharp debridement helps to create a blood-rich, uninfected wound surface in which granulation can occur. Qualified health care professionals with specific training in this care can remove tissue that's dead or loose (has a clearly visible line where viable tissue begins).

However, only a surgeon should perform surgical sharp debridement of wounds that cover very large areas or are deep and very close to vital structures, or whose edges can't be readily distinguished from viable tissues. General or regional anesthesia is required for this procedure.

Step by step

Follow standard precautions and maintain a clean or sterile field and clean or sterile technique when assisting with sharp debridement per facility policy.

1 **Administer an analgesic, as ordered.**
Give an oral drug 20 minutes before debridement, or an I.V. analgesic immediately before the procedure. Apply topical analgesics at least 15 minutes before debridement.

2 **Assist the qualified health care professional as needed.**
Provide assistance as the QHP lifts the edges of eschar, holds necrotic tissue taut with sterile forceps, and cuts dead tissue from the wound. Irrigate the wound as necessary.

3 **Apply pressure to bleeding tissues.**
If bleeding occurs, apply gentle pressure with sterile 4″ × 4″ gauze pads.

4 **Treat and dress the site as ordered.**
Apply topical medications and replace and secure the dressing, as ordered.

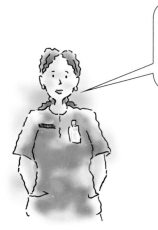

Healthy tissue

> In debridement, dead tissue is removed, which exposes healthy tissue and increases the size of the wound.

Understanding biologic debridement

Maggot therapy

Maggot therapy is a type of biological therapy in which live, sterilized, medicinal *Lucilia sericata* (green bottle fly) maggots are placed in a wound every 2 to 3 days, either directly or in a saclike device. The maggots secrete a proteinase enzyme that helps degrade necrotic tissue and digest bacteria, which promotes healing in wounds with resistant microorganism strains. The maggots also stimulate formation of granulation tissue. Although it is cost-effective and usually painless, some patients cannot tolerate the maggot movement under the bandage.

Maggot larva

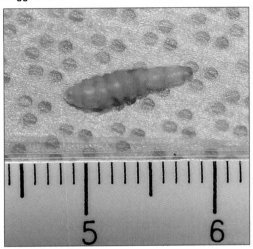

Steps
- Clean the treatment area with normal saline solution.
- Place 5 to 10 sterile maggots per square centimeter of the wound.
Protect periwound skin with a barrier cream or barrier wafer, as there may be a large amount of exudate.
- Immediately cover the wound with an appropriate dressing, see manufacturer suggestions as maggots must be able to breathe.
- Check the dressing every 6 hours for drainage, and reinforce as needed.
- Remove the maggots after therapy, usually by suctioning into a canister of alcohol.

Contraindications for patients
- with life-threatening wounds
- who would suffer psychological stress from the therapy
- with bleeding abnormalities
- with deep-tracking wounds.

Leech therapy

In leech therapy, which is sometimes used after reattachment surgery and transplantation surgery, medical leeches (*Hirudo medicinalis*) are applied to wounds to effectively:

- relieve venous congestion
- create a puncture that bleeds
- anesthetize the wound
- prevent blood clotting
- dilate vessels to increase blood flow.

Leech therapy works because leech saliva contains hirudin, a thrombin inhibitor; hyaluronidase, which helps spread the saliva and has antibiotic properties; a histamine-like vasodilator to promote local bleeding; and a local anesthetic.

Steps

- Wash the area with soap and water and then rinse it with distilled, nonchlorinated water.
- While wearing gloves, attach the leech, directing the head toward the therapy site.
- Cover the treatment area with gauze to prevent the leech from migrating to another site.
- Monitor the site every 15 minutes.
- After therapy, remove the leech by placing a small amount of alcohol, saline solution, or vinegar on a pad or a cotton swab and stroking the head of the leech until it detaches. *Note*: Do not pull the leech.

Leech anatomy

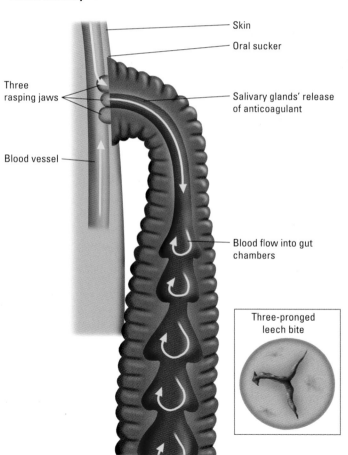

Skin

Oral sucker

Three rasping jaws

Salivary glands' release of anticoagulant

Blood vessel

Blood flow into gut chambers

Three-pronged leech bite

Documenting wound care

Documentation checklist

When documenting wound care, be sure to include:

- ☑ date, time, and type of wound care performed
- ☑ amount of soiled dressing and packing removed
- ☑ type, color, consistency, and amount of drainage
- ☑ wound appearance (size, condition of margins, presence of necrotic tissue)
- ☑ presence of odor
- ☑ presence and location of drains
- ☑ additional procedures, such as irrigation, packing, or application of a topical medication
- ☑ type and amount of new dressing or pouch applied
- ☑ patient's tolerance of the procedure.

Document special or detailed wound care instructions and pain management steps on the care plan. Also, record the amount of drainage on the intake and output sheet.

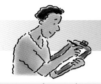

Take note

Documenting wound care

05/12/18	1430	Dressing removed from abdominal
		incision. A 2-cm round area of se-
		rosanguineous drainage noted on
		dressing. No odor noted. Incision
		well approximated except for 1.5-cm
		area at distal end of incision.
		Wound culture obtained and sent
		to lab. Incision cleaned with ster-
		ile NSS and disposable negative
		pressure therapy dressing applied.
		Pt. tolerated with 2/10 pain rating
		during dressing application. Pain
		subsided after dressing completed.
		—— David Stevens, RN

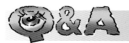

Matchmaker

Match the wound cleaning technique shown with the proper wound type for which it's used.

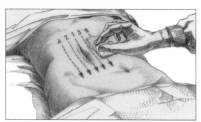

A. Circular wound

B. Linear wound

1. _____

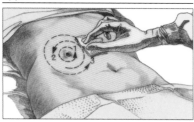

2. _____

Show and tell

State which wound care procedure is illustrated here and explain why this method is used.

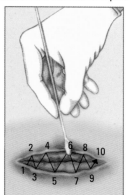

_____

_____

_____

_____

_____

Answers: Matchmaker 1. B, 2. A; Show and tell. This illustration shows culturing using the 10-point method. The 10-point method is used to ensure all possible areas of infection have been swabbed.

Selected References

Atkin, L. (2014). Understanding methods of wound debridement. *British Journal of Nursing, 23*(Suppl. 12), S10–S15.

Bryant, R. A., & Nix, D. P. (Eds.). (2012). *Acute & chronic wounds: Current management concepts.* St. Louis, MO: Elsevier Health Sciences.

Clean vs. sterile dressing techniques for management of chronic wounds: A fact sheet. (2012). *Journal of Wound, Ostomy and Continence Nursing, 39*(2S), S30–S34.

Doughty, D., & McNichol, L. (2016). *Wound, Ostomy, and Continence Nurses Society core curriculum: Wound management.* Philadelphia: Wolters Kluwer.

Griffin, J. (2014). What nurses need to know about the application of larval therapy. *Journal of Community Nursing, 28*(2), 58–62.

Haesler, E., & White, W. (2017). Minimising wound-related pain: A discussion of traditional wound dressings and topical agents used in low-resource communities. *Wound Practice and Research, 25*(3), 138–144.

Madhok, B. M., Vowden, K., & Vowden, P. (2013). New techniques for wound debridement. *International Wound Journal, 10*(3), 247–251.

Robbins, J. M., & Dillon, J. (2015). Evidence-based approach to advanced wound care products. *Journal of the American Podiatric Medical Association, 105*(5), 456–467. doi:10.7547/14-089.

Thomas, G. W., et al. (2009). Mechanisms of delayed wound healing by commonly used antiseptics. *Journal of Trauma Injury, Infection, and Critical Care, 66*(1), 82–90.

Chapter 5

Acute wounds

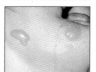
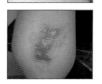

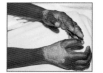

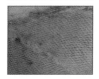
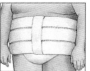
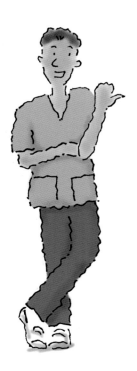

Burns

Burns are tissue injuries that result from contact with thermal, chemical, or electrical sources or from friction or exposure to the sun. They can cause cellular skin damage and a systemic response that leads to altered body function. A major burn affects every body system and organ, usually requiring painful treatment and a long period of rehabilitation. Severity is determined by total body surface burned and the depth of the burns.

Types of burns

First degree

A first-degree burn causes localized injury or destruction to the skin's epidermis by direct contact (such as a chemical spill) or indirect contact (such as sunlight).

Signs and symptoms

 Localized pain

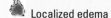 Localized edema

Erythema (usually without blisters)

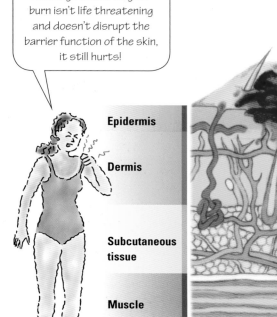

> Although a first-degree burn isn't life threatening and doesn't disrupt the barrier function of the skin, it still hurts!

Epidermis

Dermis

Subcutaneous tissue

Muscle

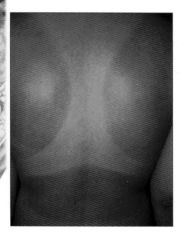

Second degree

Second-degree burns are subclassified as either **SUPERFICIAL** partial-thickness burns or **DEEP** partial-thickness burns.

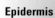

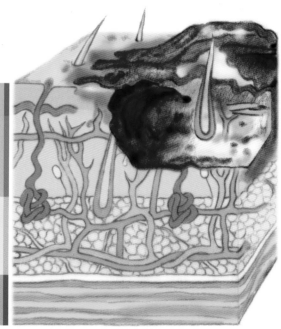

Epidermis

Dermis

Subcutaneous tissue

Muscle

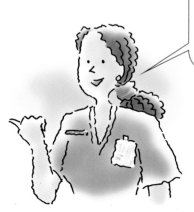

This first-degree burn resulted from sunburn. Notice the localized erythema and absence of blisters characteristic of first-degree burns.

In **SUPERFICIAL** partial-thickness burns:

- 🔥 epidermis and some dermis are destroyed
- 🔥 thin-walled, fluid-filled blisters develop within minutes of the injury
- 🔥 nerve endings become exposed to the air as blisters break
- 🔥 pain and tactile response remain intact
- 🔥 barrier function of the skin is lost
- 🔥 epithelial repair occurs within 14 days
- 🔥 no scarring occurs.

In **DEEP** partial-thickness burns:

- 🔥 epidermis and dermis are involved
- 🔥 blisters develop
- 🔥 mild-to-moderate edema and pain occur
- 🔥 damaged area may have a white, waxy appearance
- 🔥 hair follicles remain intact, so hair can regrow
- 🔥 sensory neurons undergo extensive destruction
- 🔥 healing takes greater than 14 days.

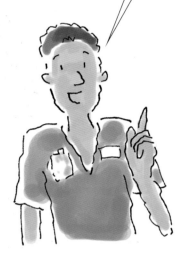

This photo shows a child with a superficial partial-thickness sunburn. Note the thin-walled, fluid-filled blisters.

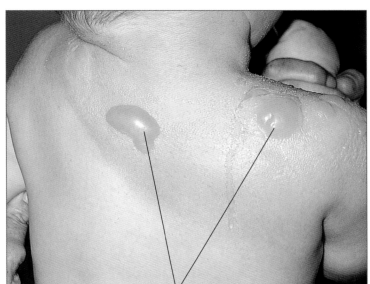

Thin-walled blisters

Here's another example of a superficial partial-thickness burn.

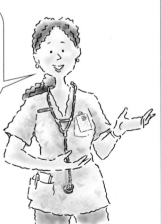

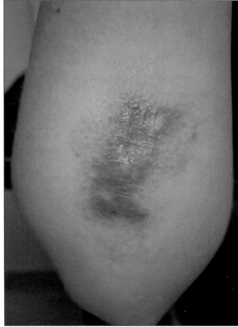

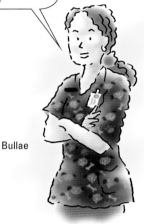

This photo shows a deep partial-thickness burn. Note the white, waxy appearance. In this instance, the large bullae will most likely be ruptured.

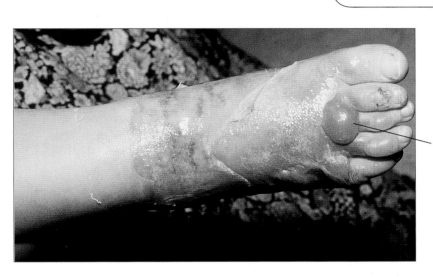

Bullae

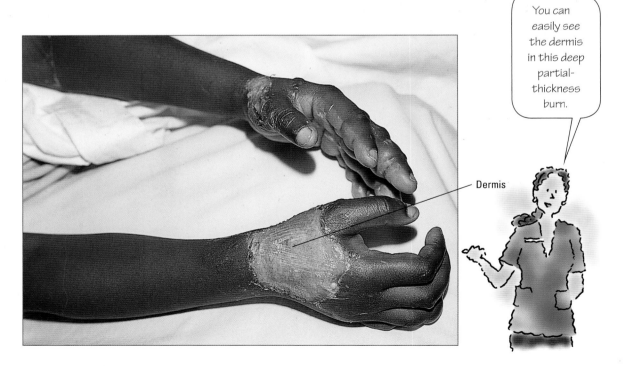

You can easily see the dermis in this deep partial-thickness burn.

Dermis

Third degree

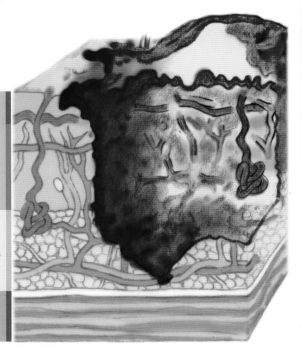

Epidermis

Dermis

Subcutaneous tissue

Muscle

Also known as *full-thickness burns*, these burns:

🔥 extend through the epidermis and dermis and into the subcutaneous tissue layer

🔥 may involve muscle, bone, and interstitial tissues

🔥 may have a white, brown, or black leathery appearance without blisters

🔥 may reveal thrombosed vessels (due to destruction of skin elasticity)

🔥 cause fluids and protein to shift from capillary to interstitial spaces within hours, causing edem

🔥 trigger an immediate immunologic response, making burn wound sepsis a potential threat.

A third-degree burn results in an increased calorie demand, which increases the patient's metabolic rate.

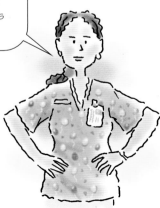

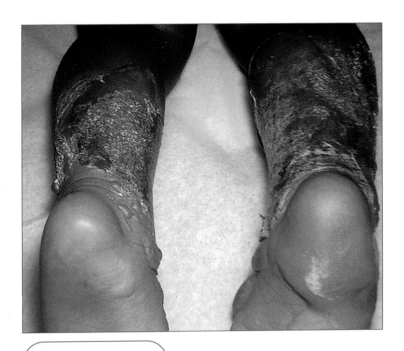

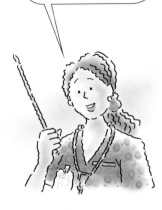

The full-thickness burns shown in this photo resulted from being scalded in a bathtub.

The black, leathery skin and absence of blisters over this hand and wrist are characteristic of third-degree burns. Notice the escharotomy performed due to circumferential eschar that can compromise circulation of the tissue underneath.

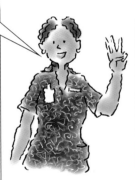

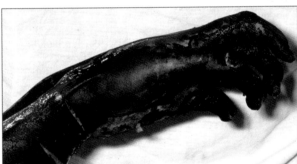

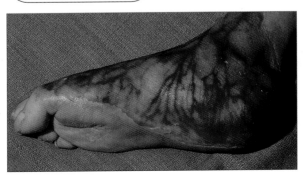

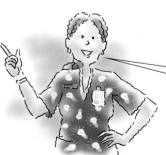

Note the thrombosed blood vessels visible in this third-degree burn of the foot.

Electrical burns

Electrical burns usually result from contact with faulty electrical wiring and cords or high-voltage power lines.

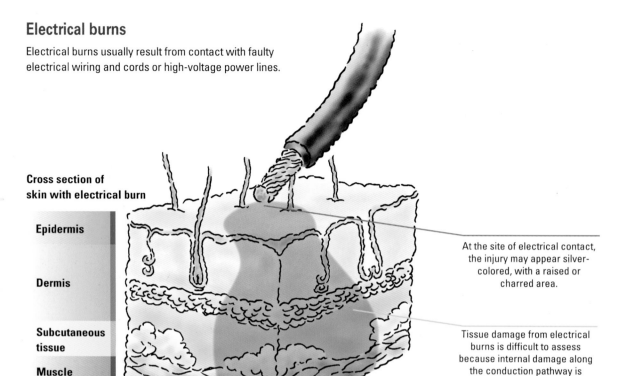

Cross section of skin with electrical burn

Epidermis

Dermis

Subcutaneous tissue

Muscle

At the site of electrical contact, the injury may appear silver-colored, with a raised or charred area.

Tissue damage from electrical burns is difficult to assess because internal damage along the conduction pathway is commonly greater than the surface burn indicates.

• Assess cardiac rhythm for life-threatening arrhythmias.
• Monitor the patient's electrolytes and urine for myoglobin since electrolyte disturbances and kidney failure can develop from the release of muscle fibers and chemicals into the bloodstream.

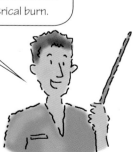

The person in this photo tried to stop a fall from a ladder by grasping a high-voltage electrical line, resulting in electrocution and an electrical burn.

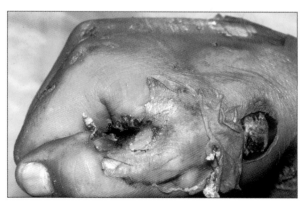

Estimating the extent of burns

Rule of Nines

You can quickly estimate the extent of an adult patient's burn by using the rule of nines. This method quantifies body surface area (BSA) in multiples of nine, giving the method its name.

To use this method, mentally assess your patient's burns according the body charts below. Add the corresponding percentages for each body section burned. Use the total—a rough estimate of the extent of the burn—to calculate initial fluid replacement needs.

> Because BSA varies with age, you'll use the rule of nines to estimate the extent of an adult patient's burns and the Lund-Browder classification to estimate the extent of an infant's or a child's burns.

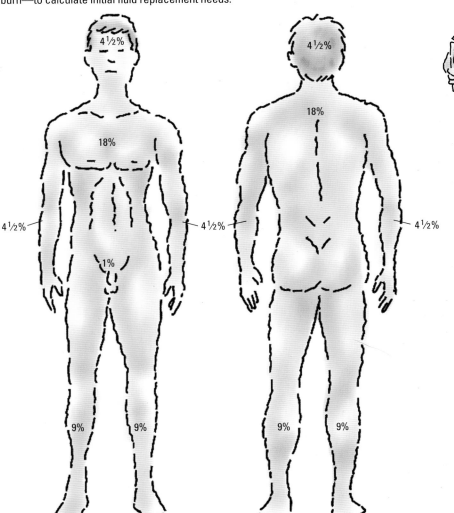

Lund-Browder classification

The rule of nines isn't accurate for infants or children because their body shapes, and therefore BSA, differ from those of adults. For example, an infant's head accounts for about 17% of total BSA, compared with 7% for an adult. Children have a higher BSA to body mass ratio so fluid losses are proportionally higher.

   Instead, use the Lund-Browder classification (shown below) to determine burn size for infants and children.

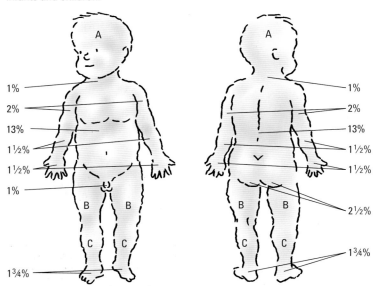

Percentage of burned body surface by age

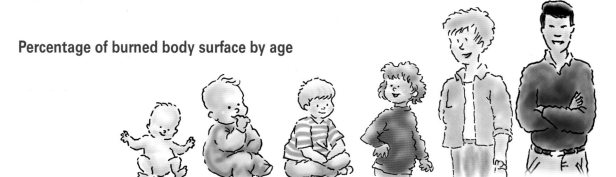

	At birth	0 to 1 year	1 to 4 years	5 to 9 years	10 to 15 years	Adult
A: Half of head	9¹/₂%	8¹/₂%	6¹/₂%	5¹/₂%	4¹/₂%	3¹/₂%
B: Half of one thigh	2³/₄%	3¹/₄%	4%	4¹/₄%	4¹/₂%	4³/₄%
C: Half of one leg	2¹/₂%	2¹/₂%	2¹/₄%	3%	3¹/₄%	3¹/₂%

Burn management

Cleanse the burns with cool running water. Do not use ice or cold water. Use mild antibacterial soap. If less than 10% BSA, use moistened NS gauze dressing. If greater than 10%, use clean, dry sheets and keep patient warm. Determine tetanus immunization status.

> Goals are to stabilize patient, control bacteria, prevent desiccation of burn, remove necrotic tissue, manage pain, and preserve function.

Comparing topical dressings

Type	Description and uses	Nursing considerations
Silver sulfadiazine 1% (antibacterial)	Apply in thick layer 1 to 2 times a day Cover with light dressing. Cleanse burn with each dressing change.	Do not use in sulfa allergy or pregnancy.
Mafenide acetate Sulfamylon (topical antibacterial)	Apply 3 to 4 times a day. Leave open to air.	Softens eschar to help debride. Use with extreme caution in sulfa allergy.
Bacitracin (topical antibacterial)	Apply 3 to 4 times a day.	Often used on the face.
Silver impregnated (absorptive, antibacterial) For example, Aquacel Ag, Acticoat Impregnated nonadherent (Xeroform, petrolatum)	Decrease dressing frequency and pain. Useful for partial-thickness wounds. Maintains moist environment. Follow manufacturer's instructions for dressing change frequency. Cut to size of wound.	Conforms to body.

Biological burn dressings

Biological dressings provide a temporary protective covering for burn wounds and clean granulation tissue. They also temporarily secure fresh skin grafts and protect graft donor sites.

In addition to stimulating new skin growth, biological dressings act like normal skin: They reduce heat loss, block infection, and minimize fluid, electrolyte, protein losses and decrease pain.

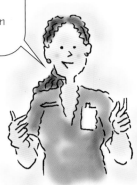

Comparing biological dressings

Type	Description and uses	Nursing considerations
Cadaver (organic, homograft or allograft)	• Applied in the operating room or at the bedside to debrided, wounds • Available as fresh cryopreserved homografts in tissue banks nationwide • Provides temporary protection, especially to granulation tissue after excision or escharotomy • May be used in some patients as a test graft for autografting	• Observe for exudate. • Watch for signs of rejection.
Pigskin (organic, heterograft or xenograft)	• Applied in the operating room or at the bedside • Comes fresh or frozen in rolls or sheets • Can cover and protect debrided wounds, mesh autografts, clean (eschar free) partial-thickness burns, and exposed tendons	• Reconstitute frozen form with normal saline solution 30 minutes before use. • Watch for signs of rejection. • Cover with gauze dressing or leave exposed to air, as ordered.
Amniotic membrane (organic, homograft)	• Human-derived collagen and growth factor • Bacteriostatic condition doesn't require antimicrobials • May be used to protect or heal partial-thickness burns or prepare site before autografting or instead of a skin graft • Applied by the qualified health care professional to clean wounds only	• Cut to size and applied to the wound. Change the membrane every 48 hours. • Cover the membrane to maintain a moist wound environment. • If you apply a gauze dressing, per manufacturer directions.
Biobrane (biosynthetic membrane)	• Made of silicone membrane bonded to nylon mesh. Available in sterile, prepackaged sheets in various sizes and in glove form for hand burns • Used to cover donor graft sites, superficial partial-thickness burns excised with or without meshed autograft. • Provides significant pain relief, decreases water vapor loss • Applied by the nurse	• Designed for one time use. Check after 24 to 36 hours for adherence then leave the membrane in place for 3 to 14 days, possibly longer. • Transparent so allows assessment of burn.

Skin grafts

Skin grafting consists of taking healthy tissue—from either the patient (autograft) or a donor (allograft)—and applying it to an area damaged by burns, traumatic injury, or surgery.

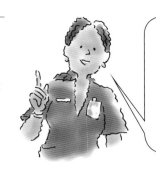

Keep in mind that a patient who has received an autograft requires care for two wounds: one at the graft site and one at the donor site.

Types of skin grafts

A burn patient may receive split-thickness grafts, full-thickness grafts, or both.

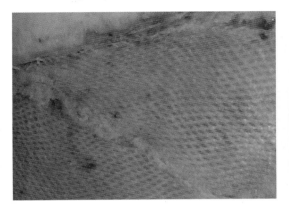
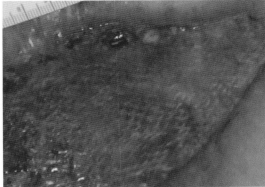

Keys to a successful skin graft

✔ Clean wound granulation with adequate vascularization

✔ Complete contact of the graft with the wound bed

✔ Maintenance of sterile technique to prevent infection

✔ Adequate graft immobilization until the graft "takes" or 5 to 7 days. Elevate extremity if indicated

✔ Monitor dressing condition, leave in place until surgeon directs to change

Common dressings used are impregnated nonadherent layer with gauze pressure dressing or negative pressure wound therapy.

Split-thickness grafts
• Include the epidermis and part of the dermis.
• Commonly used to cover open burns. Cannot be used directly over bone, tendon, or cartilage.
• May be applied as a sheet (usually on the face or neck for cosmetic purposes).
• May also be applied as a mesh (usually on extensive full-thickness burns). Meshing stretches the skin and allows coverage of a large area with a small piece of skin.
• Usually "takes" in 3 to 5 days.

Full-thickness skin grafts
• Include the epidermis and the entire dermis
• Contain hair follicles, sweat glands, and sebaceous glands
• Usually used for small deep burns as a sheet or a flap graft.

Common donor skin graft sites

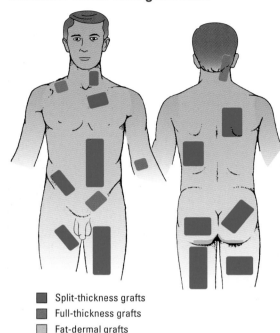

- ■ Split-thickness grafts
- ■ Full-thickness grafts
- □ Fat-dermal grafts

The donor site needs scrupulous care to prevent infection, which could cause the site to become a full-thickness wound.

Caring for a donor site

In autografting, tissue is removed from the patient's body using a dermatome, an instrument that cuts uniform, split-thickness skin portions (shown below). Consequently, the donor site is a partial-thickness wound, which may bleed, drain, and cause pain. Depending on the graft's thickness, tissue may be obtained from the donor site again in as few as 10 days.

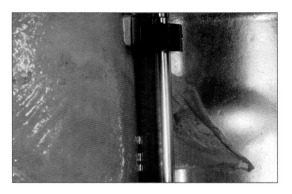

Usually, a moisture vapor–permeable dressing (transparent film dressing) or semiocclusive gauze, such as Vaseline or xeroform gauze, is applied postoperatively to protect new epithelial proliferation. Some of these partial-thickness wounds can be covered with disposable NPWT devices, which will manage drainage and protect site during healing.

Dressing the wound

- Wash your hands and put on sterile gloves.
- Remove the outer gauze dressings within 24 hours. Inspect the semiocclusive gauze dressing for signs of infection; then leave it open to the air to speed drying and healing. If using a film dressing, follow the surgeon's instructions. Reinforce with gauze if needed for leakage.
- Apply a skin emollient daily to completely healed donor sites to keep skin tissue pliable, to remove crusts, and to decrease itching.

Evacuating fluid from a sheet graft

When small pockets of fluid (called *blebs*) accumulate beneath a sheet graft, a qualified health care professional will need to evacuate the fluid using a sterile scalpel and sterile cotton-tipped applicators. Be prepared to assist, as needed.

1 The qualified health care professional will carefully perforate the center of the bleb with the scalpel.

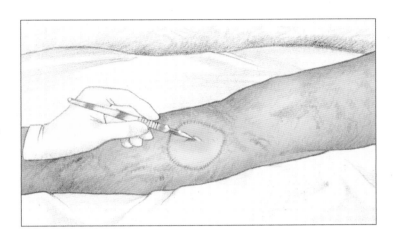

2 Then the fluid will be gently expressed with the cotton-tipped applicators.

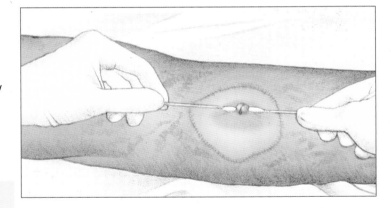

 Fluid should never be expressed by rolling the bleb to the edge of the graft. This disturbs healing in other areas.

Understanding compartment syndrome

In compartment syndrome, edema or bleeding increases pressure within a muscle compartment (arm or leg) to the point that circulation (both arterial inflow and venous outflow) to muscles and nerves within the compartment is impaired. It can occur as a result of burns, direct injury and pressure, fractures, and snake envenomation. This condition is limb threatening and requires immediate intervention.

Symptoms

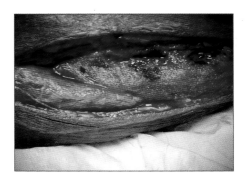

- Intense, deep, throbbing pain that doesn't improve with analgesia
- Numbness and tingling distal to the affected muscle
- Absent peripheral pulses in the affected extremity
- Pallor or mottling of the affected area
- Decreased movement, muscle strength, and sensation in the affected extremity.

Treatments

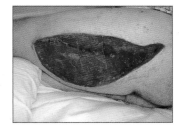

- Positioning of the affected extremity at heart level
- Removal of constrictive clothing and dressings
- Analgesics
- Neurovascular status monitoring to detect changes in circulation and nerve function
- Intracompartmental pressure monitoring and Doppler ultrasound to assess blood flow
- Emergency fasciotomy to allow muscle to expand and decrease compartment pressure
- Wound management after fasciotomy focuses on maintaining a moist wound environment. Gauze dressings or negative pressure wound therapy are used until edema resolves and granulation occurs over visible muscle. Then the wound is closed or skin graft is placed.

Surgical wounds

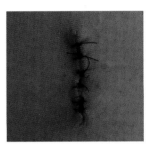

Never remove a surgical dressing without an order. Some dressings put pressure on the wound; others keep skin grafts intact. It takes up to 48 hours for the skin barrier to form.

Acute surgical wounds are uncomplicated breaks in the skin that result from surgery. In an otherwise healthy individual, these types of wounds typically heal without incident. Surgical wounds heal by three methods:

Primary intention: wound edges are approximated and secured.

Secondary intention: skin edges are not closed. Dressings are used to absorb drainage and promote healing. Used if infection is present. Wound heals by forming granulation tissue from the bottom out.

Third intention, or delayed primary closure, occurs when a contaminated wound is left open until contamination and inflammation resolve, and then closed by primary intention (this usually occurs after several days).

Assessment
First check the outside...

✔ Is the dressing stained?
- Estimate drainage quantity.
- Note its color, consistency, and odor.

✔ Does the patient have a drainage device?
- Record the amount of drainage.
- Note the color of the drainage.
- Ensure that the device is patent, secure, and free from kinks.

✔ Does the patient have an ostomy (urostomy, colostomy, ileostomy)?
- Describe the output, color, location of the stoma, security of the pouching system, and peristomal skin.

... then go under cover

✔ Is a healing ridge present?
- Are there signs and symptoms of infection, such as redness, warmth, and edema along the incision line and in the surrounding area; localized pain and tenderness; fever; pus or exudate from the incision; separation of suture line? Report these to the surgeon.

Warning!
Wound infection is the most common surgical wound complication and the second most common infection type that occurs during hospitalization.

Postoperative leg wound infection

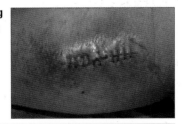

Definition: Healing ridge
"Palpable ridge that forms on each side of the wound during normal wound healing. It results from a buildup of collagen fibers, which begins to form during the inflammatory phase of wound healing and peaks during the proliferation phase (approximately 5 to 9 days postoperatively). Ridges typically fail to develop because of mechanical strain on the wound."

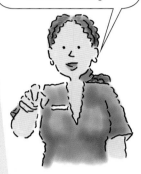

What to teach your patient about surgical wound care?

☑ Signs and symptoms of wound infection to report immediately

☑ Procedure for taking an accurate temperature reading

☑ Proper wound care, such as keeping the incision clean and dry, proper hand washing technique, and supplies and methods used to clean the wound

☑ Wound dressings, including the type, places to obtain them, and proper application

☑ Types and levels of permissible activity, such as lifting restrictions (if applicable), restrictions on bathing, smoking cessation, and expectations for returning to work

☑ Encourage good dietary intake, especially protein, to promote healing

☑ Follow-up appointments

> Being a good surgical sleuth means never going it alone. Train the patient/caregiver to care for the wound and to monitor healing.

Wound closure

The severity and location of a wound determines the type of material used to close it. Newer technologies such as skin adhesives and negative pressure wound therapy designed for closed incisions are available to enhance healing.

Topical skin adhesives

Topical skin adhesives, such as Dermabond, are applied to the approximated incision and form a strong flexible bond to the skin. The film stays in place for 5 to 10 days. It is commonly used on facial lacerations and trocar puncture sites from laparoscopic procedures. Instruct the patient that he or she may shower and then pat the area dry gently. The patient should not swim, soak, or scrub the wound until the Dermabond falls off.

Adhesive closures

Adhesive closures, such as Steri-Strips or butterfly closures, may be used to close small wounds with scant drainage or to provide continued reinforcement after suture or staple removal. Apply 1/8″ apart to clean and dry skin. Do not apply under pressure to avoid blisters.

Steri-Strips

Steri-Strips are thin strips of sterile, non-woven tape. They're a primary means of closing small wounds or holding a wound closed after suture/staple removal.

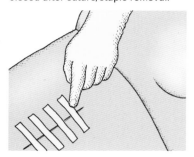

Butterfly closures

Butterfly closures consist of two sterile, waterproof adhesive strips linked by a narrow, nonadhesive "bridge." They're used to hold small wounds closed after a laceration to promote healing after suture removal.

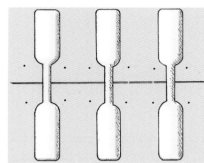

Sutures

Surgeons usually use sutures. If cosmetic results aren't an issue, the surgeon may choose to use skin staples or clips.

Suture materials
Nonabsorbable sutures
• Used to close the skin surface
• Provide strength and immobility
• Cause minimal tissue irritation
• Consist of silk, cotton, stainless steel, or nylon.

Absorbable sutures
• Broken down by the body so used when suture removal is undesirable
• Consist of:
– chromic catgut—a natural catgut treated with chromium trioxide to improve strength and prolong absorption time
– plain catgut—a material that's absorbed faster and is more likely to cause irritation than chromic catgut
– synthetic materials (such as polyglycolic acid)—materials that are replacing catgut because they're stronger, more durable, and less irritating.

Caring for and dressing surgical wounds

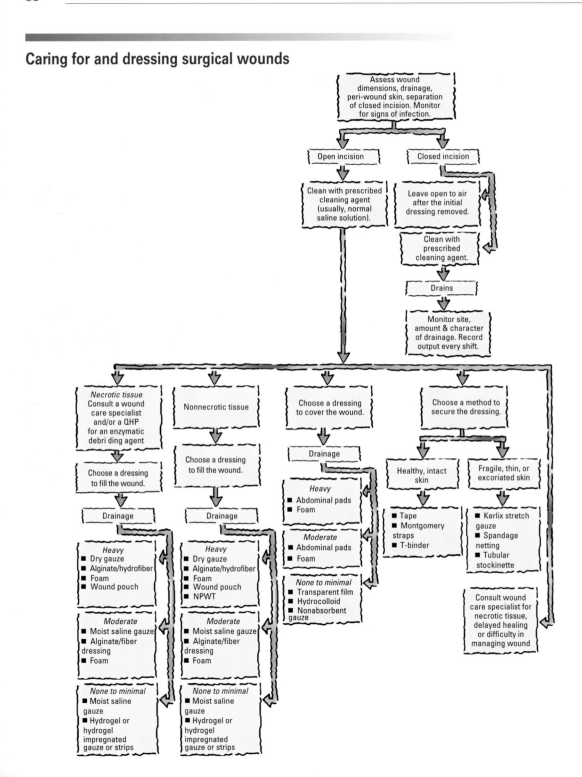

Assess wound dimensions, drainage, peri-wound skin, separation of closed incision. Monitor for signs of infection.

Open incision

Closed incision

Clean with prescribed cleaning agent (usually, normal saline solution).

Leave open to air after the initial dressing removed.

Clean with prescribed cleaning agent.

Drains

Monitor site, amount & character of drainage. Record output every shift.

Necrotic tissue Consult a wound care specialist and/or a QHP for an enzymatic debriding agent

Choose a dressing to fill the wound.

Drainage

Heavy
■ Dry gauze
■ Alginate/hydrofiber
■ Foam
■ Wound pouch

Moderate
■ Moist saline gauze
■ Alginate/fiber dressing
■ Foam

None to minimal
■ Moist saline gauze
■ Hydrogel or hydrogel impregnated gauze or strips

Nonnecrotic tissue

Choose a dressing to fill the wound.

Drainage

Heavy
■ Dry gauze
■ Alginate/hydrofiber
■ Foam
■ Wound pouch
■ NPWT

Moderate
■ Moist saline gauze
■ Alginate/fiber dressing
■ Foam

None to minimal
■ Moist saline gauze
■ Hydrogel or hydrogel impregnated gauze or strips

Choose a dressing to cover the wound.

Drainage

Heavy
■ Abdominal pads
■ Foam

Moderate
■ Abdominal pads
■ Foam

None to minimal
■ Transparent film
■ Hydrocolloid
■ Nonabsorbent gauze

Choose a method to secure the dressing.

Healthy, intact skin

■ Tape
■ Montgomery straps
■ T-binder

Fragile, thin, or excoriated skin

■ Kerlix stretch gauze
■ Spandage netting
■ Tubular stockinette

Consult wound care specialist for necrotic tissue, delayed healing or difficulty in managing wound

How to make Montgomery straps

An abdominal dressing requiring frequent changes can be secured with Montgomery straps to promote the patient's comfort and protect from MARSI (medical adhesive-related skin injury). If ready-made straps aren't available, follow these steps to make your own:

1 Cut four to six strips of 2″ to 3″ wide hypoallergenic tape of sufficient length to allow the tape to extend about 6″ (15.2 cm) beyond the wound on each side. (The length of the tape might vary according to the patient's size and the type and amount of dressing.)

2 Fold one of each strip 2″ to 3″ (5 to 7.5 cm) back on itself (sticky sides together) to form a nonadhesive tab. Then cut a small hole in the folded tab's center, close to its top edge. Make as many pairs of straps as you'll need to snugly secure the dressing.

3 Clean the patient's skin to prevent irritation. After the skin dries, apply a skin protectant. Then apply the sticky side of each tape to a skin barrier wafer or a hydrocolloid wafer, and apply the wafer directly to the skin near the dressing.

4 Thread a separate piece of gauze tie, umbilical tape, or twill tape (about 12″ [30.5 cm]) through each pair of holes in the straps, and fasten each tie as you would a shoelace. Don't stress the surrounding skin by securing the ties too tightly.

Replace Montgomery straps every 2 to 3 days or whenever they become soiled. If skin maceration occurs, place new tapes about 1″ (2.5 cm) away from irritation.

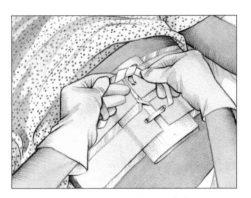

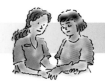

Wound care in bariatric patients

After surgery, bariatric patients experience slower wound healing because:
- Adipose tissue lacks a sufficient blood supply.
- The diaphragm doesn't descend completely, decreasing vital capacity.
- Insufficient oxygen slows digestion of bacteria by neutrophils.

They are also at increased risk for complications, such as:
- trauma (for example, the more forceful retraction needed during surgery may cause necrosis of the abdominal wall)
- infection (the difficulty level of operating on these patients lengthens the operation time, increasing the chances of contamination)
- dehiscence (excess fat and excess blood or serous fluid increase tension on the incision and wound's edges)
- hematoma.

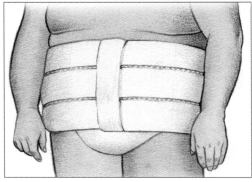

Steps to help prevent complications
- Assess the incision site and vital signs frequently.
- Use an abdominal binder over the surgical site to support the incision.
- Encourage the patient to use deep breathing and spirometry to improve oxygenation.
- Assess nutritional status and promote adequate intake of protein, carbohydrates, and vitamins.

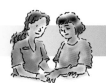

Like a retention wall, retention sutures are used to help "retain" the integrity of a wound.

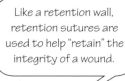

Retention sutures

Although not used exclusively for bariatric patients, retention sutures are sometimes used after surgery in overweight patients to secure a wound's edges and reinforce the suture line. They can also be used for patients who have had multiple procedures in

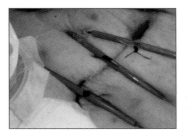

a short time or who are at high risk for wound dehiscence. Placed through the abdominal wall before the abdominal layers are closed, they provide support to deep tissue while the more superficial fascia and skin tissue heal. Monitor the entry site at the skin to prevent device-related pressure injuries. And keep the skin around these sutures clean.

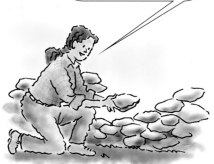

Surgical drains

Surgeons insert closed wound drains during surgery when they expect a large amount of postoperative drainage. These drains suction serosanguineous fluid from the wound site.

If a wound produces heavy drainage, the closed wound drain may be left in place for longer than 1 week. Drainage must be frequently emptied and measured to maintain maximum suction and prevent strain on the suture line. Treat the tubing exit site as an additional surgical wound. Be sure to secure the drainage device so it does not pull or become dislodged.

Purposes
- Promote healing
- Prevent swelling
- Reduce risk of infection and skin breakdown
- Minimize the need for dressing changes

Closed wound drainage system

A closed wound drain consists of perforated tubing which facilitates drainage and is connected to a portable vacuum unit. (Hemovac and Jackson-Pratt are the most commonly used drainage systems.) The distal end of the tubing lies within the wound and usually leaves the body from a site other than the primary suture line. The drain is usually sutured to the skin. Shown below is a closed wound drainage system in a postmastectomy patient.

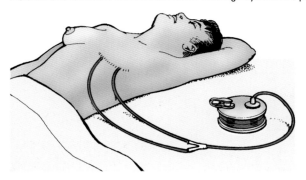

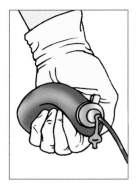

To empty the drainage, remove the plug and empty it into a graduate cylinder. To reestablish suction in a Hemovac unit, compress the drainage unit against a firm surface to expel air and, while holding it down, replace the plug with your other hand (as shown above).

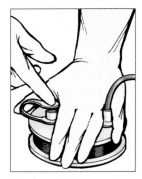

Follow a similar procedure to reestablish suction in a Jackson-Pratt bulb drain (shown above).

Surgical drain

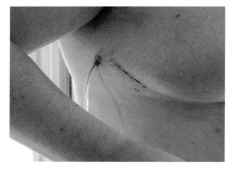

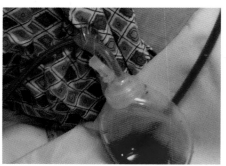

Ostomy care

A patient with a urostomy, colostomy, or ileostomy wears an external pouch over the ostomy site, usually attached with a barrier wafer. The pouch collects urine or fecal matter, helps control odor, and protects the stoma and peristomal skin. Most disposable pouching systems can be used for 3 to 7 days, unless a leak develops.

When selecting a pouching system, choose one that delivers the best adhesive seal and skin protection for that patient. Other considerations include the stoma's location and structure, consistency of the effluent, availability and cost of supplies, amount of time the patient will wear the pouch, any known adhesive allergy, and the personal preferences of the patient.

For colostomies or ileostomies, the best time to change a pouching system is first thing in the morning or 2 to 4 hours after meals, when the bowel is least active. After a few months, most patients can predict the time that's best for them.

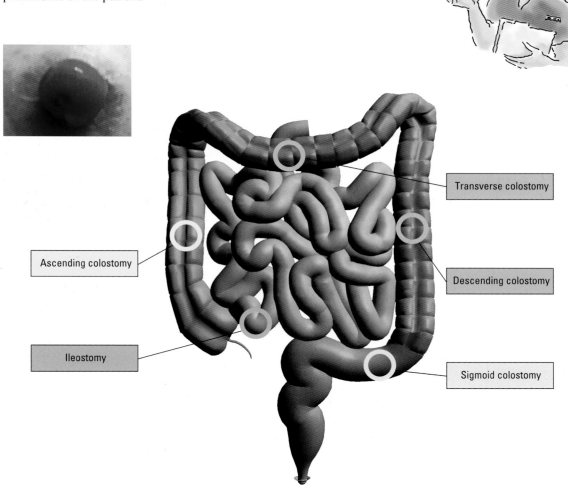

Transverse colostomy

Ascending colostomy

Descending colostomy

Ileostomy

Sigmoid colostomy

Comparing ostomy pouching systems

Manufactured in many shapes and sizes, ostomy pouches are fashioned for comfort, safety, and easy application. Some commonly available pouches are described here.

Disposable pouches

Patients who must empty their pouch often (because of diarrhea or a new colostomy or ileostomy) may prefer a one-piece, drainable, disposable pouch attached to a skin barrier. This pouch may be used permanently or temporarily, until stoma size stabilizes.

Disposable closed-end pouches, made of transparent or opaque odor-proof plastic, may come with a carbon filter for gas release. A patient with a regular bowel elimination pattern may choose this style for additional security and confidence.

A two-piece disposable drainable pouch with separate skin barrier permits frequent changes of the pouch while minimizing barrier removal.

Urostomy pouches have a spout on the end that can be connected to straight drainage for overnight or leg bag collection.

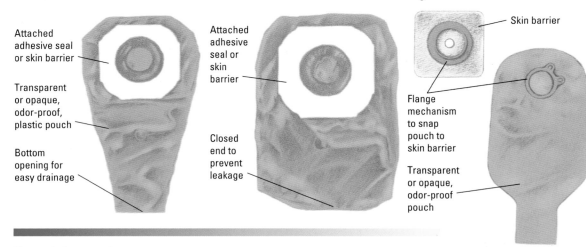

Attached adhesive seal or skin barrier

Transparent or opaque, odor-proof, plastic pouch

Bottom opening for easy drainage

Attached adhesive seal or skin barrier

Closed end to prevent leakage

Skin barrier

Flange mechanism to snap pouch to skin barrier

Transparent or opaque, odor-proof pouch

Reusable pouches

Reusable pouches come with a separate custom-made faceplate and O-ring (as shown at right). Some pouches have a pressure valve for releasing gas. The device has a 1- to 2-month life span, depending on how frequently the patient empties the pouch. It is secured to the abdomen with a belt.

Reusable equipment may benefit a patient who needs a firm faceplate, or has skin reactions to adhesives in the disposable barrier. However, many reusable ostomy pouches aren't as odor proof as the disposable pouches.

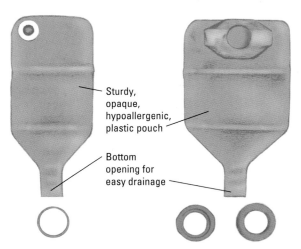

Sturdy, opaque, hypoallergenic, plastic pouch

Bottom opening for easy drainage

Applying a skin barrier and pouch

Fitting a skin barrier and ostomy pouch properly can be done in a few steps. Shown here is a two-piece pouching system with flanges, which is commonly used.

1 Measure the stoma using a measuring guide.

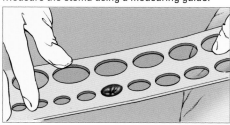

2 Trace the appropriate circle carefully on the back of the skin barrier.

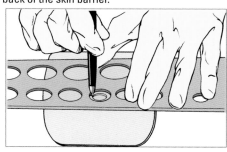

3 Cut the circular opening in the skin barrier. Bevel the edges to keep them from irritating the patient. Be sure to size the opening correctly to prevent peristomal skin breakdown (approximately 1/8″ larger than the stoma).

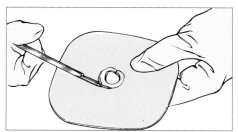

4 Remove the backing from the skin barrier. Apply a barrier ring or paste, if needed, along the edge of the circular opening.

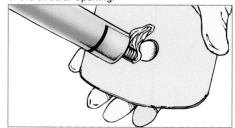

5 Center the skin barrier over the stoma, adhesive side down, and gently press it to the skin.

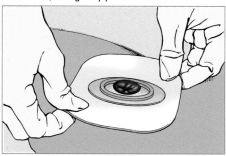

6 Gently press the pouch opening onto the ring until it snaps into place.

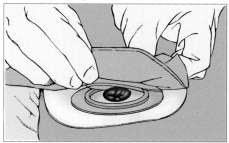

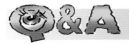

Matchmaker

Match the picture to the clinical condition

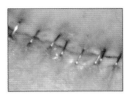

1. _____

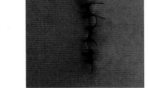

2. _____

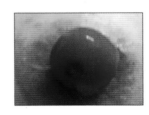

3. _____

A. stapled wound

B. normal stoma

C. healing by primary intention

D. healing by secondary intention

E. peristomal irritant dermatitis

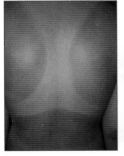

4. _____

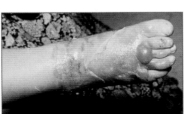

5. _____

Show and tell

Identify the type of burn shown in each of these photos.

1. _____

2. _____

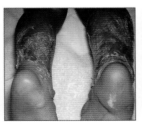

3. _____

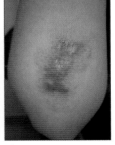

4. _____

Answers: Matchmaker 1. Normal stapled wound, 2. Wound closed by primary intention, 3. Normal stoma wound, 4. Healing by secondary intention, 5. Irritant dermatitis due to improper barrier application. *Answers: Show and tell* 1. First-degree burn, 2. Deep partial-thickness burn, 3. Third-degree burn, 4. Second-degree burn.

Selected References

Delmore, B., Cohen, J., O'Neill, D., Chu, A., Pham, V., & Chiu, E. (2017). Reducing postsurgical wound complications: A critical review. *Advances in Skin and Wound Care, 30*(6), 272–285.

Ethicon Inc. (2007). *Ethicon wound closure manual.* Somerville, NJ: Author.

Glat, P. M., & Davenport, T. (2017). Current techniques for burn reconstruction using dehydrated amnion/chorion membrane allografts as an adjunctive treatment along the reconstructive ladder. *Annals of Plastic Surgery, 78*(Suppl. 1), S14–S18.

ISBI Practice Guidelines Committee. (2016). ISBI practice guidelines for burn care. *Burns, 42,* 953–1021.

Singer, A., & Boyce, S. (2017). Burn wound healing and tissue engineering. *Journal of Burn Care and Research, 38*(3), e605–e613.

Texas EMS Trauma & Acute Care Foundation Trauma Division. (2016). *Burn clinical practice guideline.* Retrieved from http://tetaf.org/wp-content/uploads/2016/01/Burn-Practice-Guideline.pdf

Trofino, R. (2015). Nursing care of patients with burns. In L. S. Williams (Ed.), *Understanding medical surgical nursing* (5th ed.). (0-8036-4068-4, 978-0-8036-4068-9). Philadelphia, PA: F. A. Davis Company.

Warner, P., Coffee, T., & Yowler, C. (2014). Outpatient burn management. *Surgical Clinics of North America, 94,* 879–892.

Wax, M. (2017). Split thickness skin grafts. Retrieved from http://emedicine.medscape.com/article/876290-overview#a6

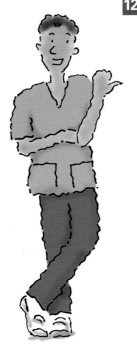

Chapter 6

Pressure injuries

Definition

Pressure injury is localized damage to the skin and underlying soft tissue usually over a bony prominence or related to a medical or other device. The injury can present as intact skin or an open ulcer and may be painful.

Causes

Pressure injuries typically occur as a result of intense and/or prolonged pressure or pressure combined with shear. Body tissues differ in their ability to tolerate pressure. This tolerance of soft tissue for pressure and shear may also be affected by microclimate, nutrition, perfusion, comorbidities, and condition of the soft tissue.

An estimated 2.5 million pressure injuries occur each year in the United States, with one-half of those being stage 2 or greater.

Understanding the pressure gradient

A V-shaped pressure gradient results from the upward force exerted by a support surface and the downward force of a bony prominence. Pressure is greatest on tissues at the apex of the gradient and lessens to the right and left of this point. This leads to deformity in the tissue and stress and strain within the tissue.

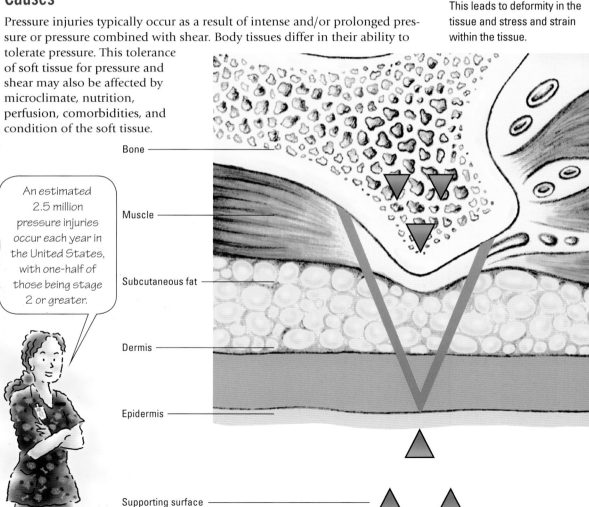

Bone

Muscle

Subcutaneous fat

Dermis

Epidermis

Supporting surface

Sitting

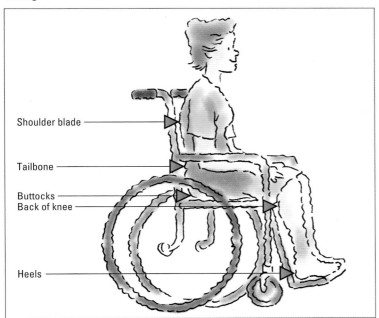

Shoulder blade

Tailbone

Buttocks
Back of knee

Heels

Lying

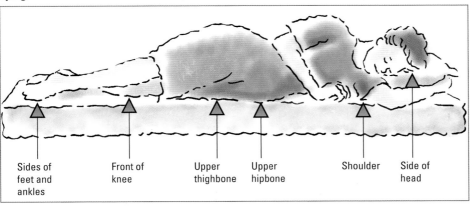

Sides of
feet and
ankles

Front of
knee

Upper
thighbone

Upper
hipbone

Shoulder

Side of
head

These illustrations show the areas most likely to develop pressure injuries.

Understanding shearing force

Shear is a mechanical force that occurs parallel, rather than perpendicular, to an area of tissue. In this illustration, gravity pulls the body down the incline of the bed. The skeleton and attached tissues move, but the skin remains stationary, held in place by friction between the skin and the bed linen. The skeleton and attached tissues actually slide within the skin, causing damage to deeper tissues. Elevating the head of the bed contributes to shear injuries.

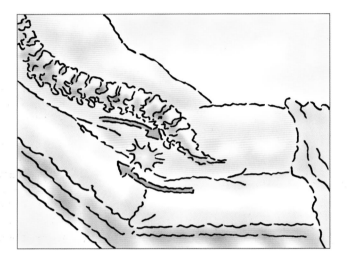

Risk factors

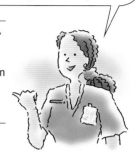

High-risk patients, whether in an institution or at home, should be assessed regularly for pressure injuries. Be sure to consider all risk factors when assessing patients.

Risk factor	Considerations
Advanced age	• Skin has less moisture and becomes more fragile as epidermal turnover slows, vascularization decreases, and skin layers adhere less securely to one another • There is less elasticity and decreased barrier function. • Older adults have less lean body mass and less subcutaneous tissue to cushion bony areas. • Underlying problems that increase pressure injury risk include poor hydration and impaired respiratory and immune systems.
Immobility	• Immobility may be the greatest risk factor for pressure injury development. • The person may be less able to move in response to pressure sensations, and body position may be changed less frequently.
Incontinence	• Incontinence increases a patient's exposure to moisture and, over time, increases risk of skin breakdown. • Urinary and fecal incontinence together can result in excessive moisture and chemical irritation.
Infection	• Compressed skin has a lower local resistance to bacterial infection. • Infection may reduce the pressure needed to cause tissue necrosis.
Low blood pressure	• Low blood pressure can lead to tissue ischemia, particularly in patients with vascular disorders. • As tissue perfusion drops, the skin is less tolerant of sustained external pressure, increasing the risk of damage from ischemia.
Malnutrition	• A strong correlation exists between poor nutrition and the development of pressure injury. • The body requires increased protein for healing; malnutrition can lead to decreased protein levels, including decreased albumin. • A direct correlation exists between pressure injury stage and the degree of hypoalbuminemia.

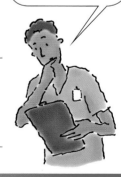

There is no one single risk factor but a complicated interplay of factors that can result in a pressure injury.

Special attention

Pressure injuries in bariatric patients

Bariatric patients are at increased risk for pressure injury development for several reasons:
• Their nutritional status might not be optimum.
• They're prone to developing protein malnutrition during metabolic stress (even though they may have excess body fat storage).
• Adipose tissue commonly has decreased vascularity.
• They may be unable to change position or move independently easily.
• The moist environment in skinfolds promotes bacterial growth, which can lead to fungal infections and decreased skin integrity.

Braden scale for predicting pressure sore risk

Tally the numbers for each subscale using the description that applies to your patient. Determine your patient's risk as follows:

- 15 to 18: At risk
- 13 to 14: Moderate risk
- 10 to 12: High risk
- 9 or below: Very high risk.

Sensory perception: Ability to respond meaningfully to pressure-related discomfort

1. Completely limited
Unresponsive (does not moan, flinch, or grasp) to painful stimuli due to diminished level of consciousness or sedation OR Limited ability to feel pain over most of body

2. Very limited
Responds only to painful stimuli. Cannot communicate discomfort except by moaning or restlessness. OR Has a sensory impairment which limits the ability to feel pain or discomfort over ½ of body.

Moisture: Degree to which skin is exposed to moisture

1. Constantly moist
Skin is kept moist almost constantly by perspiration, urine, etc. Dampness is detected every time patient is moved or turned.

2. Very moist
Skin is often, but not always moist. Linen must be changed at least once a shift.

Activity: Degree of physical activity

1. Bedfast
Confined to bed.

2. Chairfast
Ability to walk severely limited or nonexistent. Cannot bear own weight and/or must be assisted into chair or wheelchair.

Mobility: Ability to change and control body position

1. Completely immobile
Does not make even slight changes in body or extremity position without assistance.

2. Very limited
Makes occasional slight changes in body or extremity position but unable to make frequent or significant changes independently.

Nutrition: Usual food intake pattern

1. Very poor
Never eats a complete meal. Rarely eats more than 1/3 of any food offered. Eats 2 servings or less of protein (meat or dairy products) per day. Takes fluids poorly. Does not take a liquid dietary supplement. OR Is NPO and/or maintained on clear liquids or IVs for more than 5 days.

2. Probably inadequate
Rarely eats a complete meal and generally eats only about ½ of any food offered. Protein intake includes only 3 servings of meat or dairy products per day. Occasionally will take a dietary supplement. OR Receives less than optimum amount of liquid diet or tube feeding.

Friction and shear

1. Problem
Requires moderate to maximum assistance in moving. Complete lifting without sliding against sheets is impossible. Frequently slides down in bed or chair, requiring frequent repositioning with maximum assistance. Spasticity, contractures, or agitation leads to almost constant friction.

2. Potential problem
Moves feebly or requires minimum assistance. During a move skin probably slides to some extent against sheets, chair, restraints or other devices. Maintains relatively good position in chair or bed most of the time but occasionally slides down.

Patient's name _____   Evaluator's name _____

	Date of assessment		

3. Slightly limited
Responds to verbal commands but cannot always communicate discomfort or the need to be turned. OR Has some sensory impairment which limits ability to feel pain or discomfort in 1 or 2 extremities.

4. No impairment
Responds to verbal commands. Has no sensory deficit which would limit ability to feel or voice pain or discomfort.

3. Occasionally moist
Skin is occasionally moist, requiring an extra linen change approximately once a day.

4. Rarely moist
Skin is usually dry; linen only requires changing only at routine intervals.

3. Walks occasionally
Walks occasionally during day, but for very short distances, with or without assistance. Spends majority of each shift in a bed or chair.

4. Walks frequently
Walks outside room at least twice a day and inside room at least once every two hours during waking hours.

3. Slightly limited
Makes frequent though slight changes in body or extremity position independently.

4. No limitations
Makes major and frequent changes in position without assistance.

3. Adequate
Eats over half of most meals. Eats a total of 4 servings of protein (meat, dairy products) per day. Occasionally will refuse a meal, but will usually take a supplement when offered. OR Is on a tube feeding or TPN regimen which probably meets most of nutritional needs.

4. Excellent
Eats most of every meal. Never refuses a meal. Usually eats a total of 4 or more servings of meat and dairy products. Occasionally eats between meals. Does not require supplementation.

The Braden scale is the most widely used scale in the United States for determining a patient's risk of pressure injuries.

3. No apparent problem
Moves in bed and in chair independently and has sufficient muscle strength to lift up completely during move. Maintains good position in bed or chair.

Total score

Norton scale

Total the numbers from each category that describes your patient. A score of 14 or less indicates a risk of developing pressure ulcers.

Physical condition		Mental condition		Activity		Mobility		Incontinence		
Good	4	Alert	4	Ambulatory	4	Full	4	None	4	
Fair	3	Apathetic	3	Walk/help	3	Slightly limited	3	Occasional	3	**Total**
Poor	2	Confused	2	Chairbound	2	Very limited	2	Usually-urine	2	**score**
Very bad	1	Stuporous	1	Bedridden	1	Immobile	1	Urine/feces	1	

Name:	Date:					
Name:	Date:					
Name:	Date:					

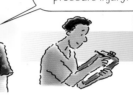

The Norton scale is another scale recommended to determine a patient's risk of pressure injury.

When to assess and reassess

How frequently you assess and reassess your patient for pressure injury risk will depend on the care setting. The Agency for Healthcare Research and Quality and the Wound, Ostomy, and Continence Nurses Society recommend the following intervals:

• Acute care: Upon admission and then daily or when the patient's condition changes. Some critical care areas complete risk assessment every shift.

• Long-term care: Upon admission and then weekly for the first 4 weeks, then monthly or whenever the patient's condition changes.

• Home health care: Upon admission and at every nursing visit.

Take note

Pressure injury documentation

Most electronic health records have options that can be selected based on your patient assessment. Here are some criteria for pressure injury documentation that are included:

Body location

Stage

Size—length x width x depth in centimeters

Tissue type—granulation, slough, eschar

Color of wound base

Periwound skin

Presence of undermining, tunneling, sinus tracts

Exudate—amount and character

Odor

Pain

Signs of infection

Status—New, improved, unchanged, deteriorating

Once your assessment is complete, be sure to document interventions and patient response. Include the following:

Topical therapy

Pressure redistribution surface(s)

Positioning schedule

Nutrition plan

Moisture management if indicated

Pain management.

Prevention

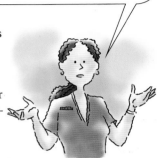

> Preventing pressure injuries—includes identifying patients at risk and taking action to minimize those risks— is a major health care goal.

Managing the intensity and duration of pressure is key to preventing pressure injuries, especially for patients with limited mobility. Other prevention strategies include reducing friction and shear, minimizing moisture, maximizing nutritional status, and controlling chronic illnesses that contribute to pressure injury development (such as diabetes). Recently, select foam dressings have been used over bony prominences in high-risk patients to prevent pressure injuries. Regular skin assessment and pressure injury risk assessment are a vital part of the prevention plan. Remember that changes in darkly pigmented skin may not be easily visible, so these patients need especially careful assessment. Notice the differences in the stage 1 pictures between the person with light vs dark complexion.

Positioning patients

All at-risk patients should have an individualized repositioning plan when in bed or chair. Even patients on a specialized support surface, or those patients with continuous lateral rotation therapy (CLRT) for respiratory issues, need to be repositioned. To position a reclining patient and turning the patient 30 degrees, use the Rule of 30 (raising the head of the bed 30 degrees, as shown below). Raising the head more than 30 degrees can cause shearing pressure. When you must raise it more (such as at mealtimes), keep the periods brief.

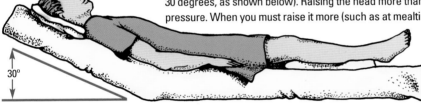

30°

When repositioning a patient from the left side to the right, make sure the weight rests on the buttock, not the hip bone. This reduces pressure on the trochanter and sacrum. The angle between the bed and an imaginary lateral line through the hips should be about 30 degrees (as shown here).

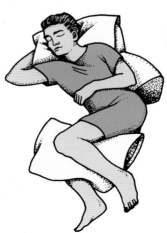

If needed, use pillows or a foam wedge to help the patient maintain the proper position. Cushion pressure points, such as the knees and shoulders, with pillows. Consider using a patient monitoring position system to assist in maintaining an appropriate turning schedule and 25- to 30-degree turn angle.

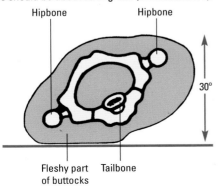

Hipbone   Hipbone

30°

Fleshy part   Tailbone
of buttocks

Pressure injury prevention algorithm

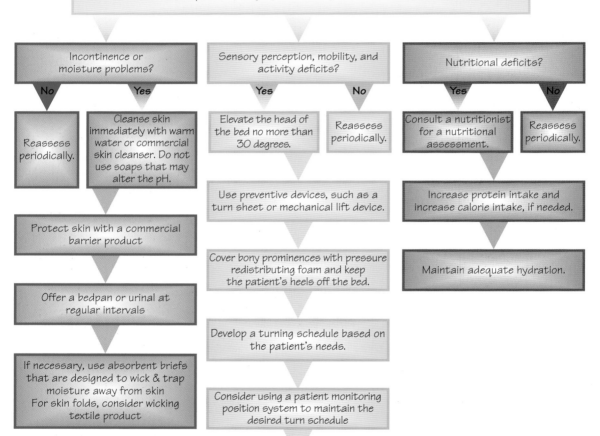

Provide patient teaching. ◄ **Yes** — **Risk for activity or mobility deficit?** — **No** ► **Reassess periodically.**

Yes

Assess pressure injury risk using an assessment tool.

Incontinence or moisture problems?

No — Reassess periodically.

Yes — Cleanse skin immediately with warm water or commercial skin cleanser. Do not use soaps that may alter the pH.

Protect skin with a commercial barrier product

Offer a bedpan or urinal at regular intervals

If necessary, use absorbent briefs that are designed to wick & trap moisture away from skin
For skin folds, consider wicking textile product

Sensory perception, mobility, and activity deficits?

Yes — Elevate the head of the bed no more than 30 degrees.

No — Reassess periodically.

Use preventive devices, such as a turn sheet or mechanical lift device.

Cover bony prominences with pressure redistributing foam and keep the patient's heels off the bed.

Develop a turning schedule based on the patient's needs.

Consider using a patient monitoring position system to maintain the desired turn schedule

Consult a wound care specialist for appropriate pressure re-distributing devices and surfaces and for further assessment.

Consult a physical therapist to help increase mobility.

Nutritional deficits?

Yes — Consult a nutritionist for a nutritional assessment.

No — Reassess periodically.

Increase protein intake and increase calorie intake, if needed.

Maintain adequate hydration.

Comparing support surface characteristics

Support surfaces are specialized devices for pressure redistribution that distribute load over the contact areas of the body. They work by managing tissue load and microclimate. Check specific product information to determine what is the best for the individualized patient's needs. And don't forget the chair cushion!

Important points:

Consider your patient's weight and the weight limitations of the surface

Many surfaces are contraindicated with unstable cervical, thoracic, or lumbar spine

Consider fall risk and bed height if the patient is restless, combative or agitated

Patients with multiple stage 2, large or multiple stage 3 or 4 pressure injuries on trunk and pelvis involving more than one turning surface should have low air loss or air-fluidized therapy.

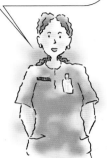

Patients need physical support to combat pressure injuries.

Braden mobility subscale scores

Braden Moisture Subscale Scores	4 or 3 No limitations or slightly limited	2 or 1 Very limited or completely immobile
4 or 3 *Rarely or occasionally moist*	Reactive CLP AMG sheepskin prevention	Reactive CLP Active with AP
2 *Very moist*	Reactive/CLP Reactive/CLP with LAL	Reactive/CLP with LAL
1 *Constantly moist*	Reactive/CLP Reactive/CLP with LAL	Reactive/CLP with LAL Reactive/CLP with AF

CLP = constant low pressure; LAL = low air loss; AP = alternating pressure; AF = air fluidized; AMG = Australian medical grade.

Reactive = provides pressure redistribution in response to an applied load (patient) by immersion and envelopment, powered or nonpowered

Active = powered surface that can change load redistribution with or without applied load (patient)

McNichol, L., Watts, C., Mackey, D., Beitz, J., & Gray, M. (2015). Identifying the right surface for the right patient at the right time: Generation and content validation of an algorithm for support surface selection. *Journal of Wound, Ostomy, and Continence Nursing, 42*(1), 19–37.

Air-fluidized therapy bed

The fluid-like surface of an air-fluidized therapy bed redistributes pressure on the skin by forcing air through beads. It conforms to the body as the patient sinks into the surface. It helps prevent pressure injuries and promote wound healing. The bed also provides the advantages of flotation without the disadvantages of instability, patient positioning difficulties, and immobility.

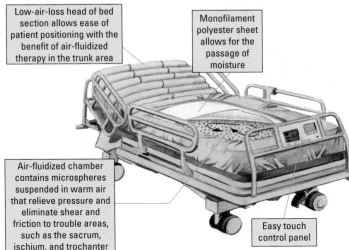

Low-air-loss head of bed section allows ease of patient positioning with the benefit of air-fluidized therapy in the trunk area

Monofilament polyester sheet allows for the passage of moisture

Air-fluidized chamber contains microspheres suspended in warm air that relieve pressure and eliminate shear and friction to trouble areas, such as the sacrum, ischium, and trochanter

Easy touch control panel

Low air loss therapy bed

Low air loss therapy beds contain segmented air cushions that inflate to help redistribute pressure on skin surfaces and to minimize shearing force during repositioning. The beds also help manage heat and humidity (microclimate) of the skin. This option can be an integrated bed system or a specialized mattress overlay that fits on regular hospital bed frames.

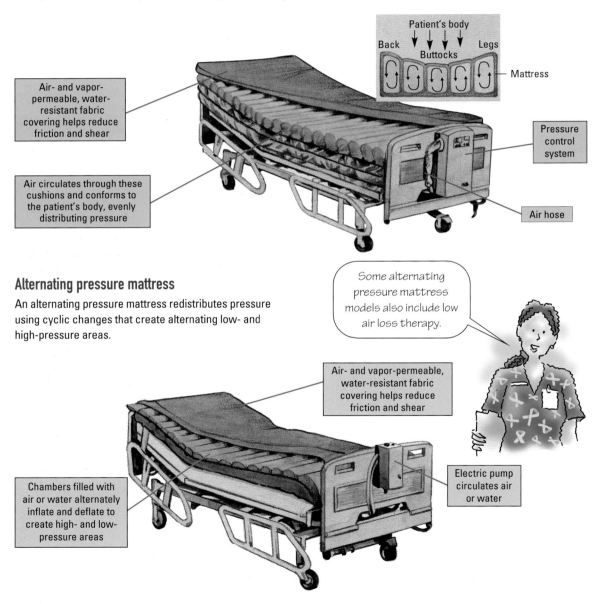

Patient's body

Back   Legs
Buttocks

Mattress

Air- and vapor-permeable, water-resistant fabric covering helps reduce friction and shear

Pressure control system

Air circulates through these cushions and conforms to the patient's body, evenly distributing pressure

Air hose

Alternating pressure mattress

An alternating pressure mattress redistributes pressure using cyclic changes that create alternating low- and high-pressure areas.

Some alternating pressure mattress models also include low air loss therapy.

Air- and vapor-permeable, water-resistant fabric covering helps reduce friction and shear

Chambers filled with air or water alternately inflate and deflate to create high- and low-pressure areas

Electric pump circulates air or water

Reactive/constant low-pressure (CLP) surface

A nonpowered or powered mattress or overlay support surface that redistributes pressure in response to the person's body weight by immersion and envelopment. This includes foam, gel, fiber, viscous fluid, static air or water, or bead-filled mattress.

Using a hydraulic lift

Using a hydraulic lift to transfer an immobile or obese patient reduces the effects of shear and friction on the skin—a key strategy of pressure injury prevention. It is also safer for the caregivers. These general guidelines will help you to transfer your patient safely and comfortably. Be sure to follow the manufacturer's instructions.

1 After placing the patient in a supine position in the center of the sling, position the hydraulic lift above the patient (as shown below). Then attach the chains to the hooks on the sling.

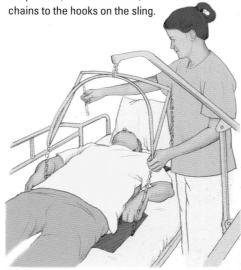

2 Turn the lift handle clockwise to raise the patient to the sitting position. If the patient's positioned properly, continue to raise until the patient's suspended just above the bed.

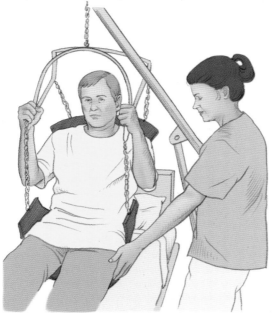

3 After positioning the patient above the wheelchair, turn the lift handle counterclockwise to lower the patient onto the seat. When the chains become slack, stop turning and unhook the sling from the lift.

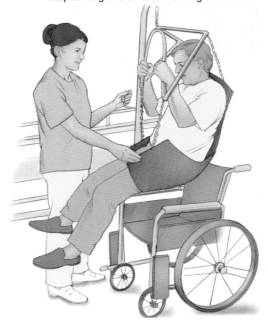

> The Pressure Ulcer Scale for Healing (PUSH) tool can help you monitor, reassess, and document pressure injuries.

Assessment

Assess pressure injuries weekly. A well-vascularized pressure injury without infection should show signs of healing within 2 weeks. If not, reevaluate the care plan.

PUSH tool

Patient's name: _____ Patient ID #: _____

Ulcer location: _____ Date: _____

Directions
Observe and measure the pressure ulcer. Categorize the ulcer with respect to surface area, exudate, and type of wound tissue. Record a subscore for each of the ulcer characteristics. Add the subscores to obtain the total score. A comparison of total scores measured over time provides an indication of the improvement or deterioration in pressure ulcer healing.

Length × width — Subscore

0 cm^2	1 < 0.3 cm^2	2 0.3 to 0.6 cm^2	3 0.7 to 1 cm^2	4 1.1 to 2 cm^2	5 2.1 to 3 cm^2
	6 3.1 to 4 cm^2	7 4.1 to 8 cm^2	8 8.1 to 12 cm^2	9 12.1 to 24 cm^2	10 > 24 cm^2

Exudate amount — Subscore

0 None	1 Light	2 Moderate	3 Heavy	—	—

Tissue type — Subscore

0 Closed	1 Epithelial tissue	2 Granulation tissue	3 Slough	4 Necrotic tissue	—

Total score

Length × width
Measure the greatest length (head to toe) and the greatest width (side to side) using a centimeter ruler. Multiply these two measurements (length × width) to obtain an estimate of surface area in square centimeters (cm^2). Don't guess! Always use a centimeter ruler and always use the same method each time you measure.

Exudate amount
Estimate the amount of exudate (drainage) present after removing the dressing and before applying any topical agent to the ulcer. Estimate as none, light, moderate, or heavy.

Tissue type
This refers to the types of tissue in the wound bed. Score as a 4 if you note necrotic tissue. Score as a 3 if you observe

slough but no necrotic tissue. Score a clean wound that contains granulation tissue as a 2. Score a superficial wound that's reepithelializing as a 1. When the wound is closed, score it as a 0. The following guide describes each tissue type:
4—Necrotic tissue (eschar): Black, brown, or tan tissue that adheres firmly to the wound bed or ulcer edges and may be either firmer or softer than surrounding tissue
3—Slough: Yellow or white tissue that adheres to the ulcer bed in strings or thick clumps or is mucinous
2—Granulation tissue: Pink or beefy red tissue with a shiny, moist, granular appearance
1—Epithelial tissue: For superficial ulcers, new pink or shiny tissue (skin) that grows in from the edges or as islands on the ulcer surface
0—Closed or resurfaced: Completely covered wound with epithelium (new skin).

Staging

Pressure injury staging reflects the depth and extent of tissue involvement. The classification system developed by the National Pressure Ulcer Advisory Panel (NPUAP) is the most widely used system for staging pressure injuries. The NPUAP recently redefined its pressure injury stages as shown below and added two new stages for device-related and mucosal membrane–related pressure injuries.

The wording has been changed from "ulcer" to "injury" to better define the physiologic process.

Deep tissue injury

Deep tissue injury is characterized by intact or nonintact skin with localized area of persistent non-blanchable deep red, maroon, purple discoloration or epidermal separation revealing a dark wound bed or blood-filled blister. Pain and temperature change often precede skin color changes. Discoloration may appear differently in darkly pigmented skin. This injury results from intense and/or prolonged pressure and shear forces at the bone-muscle interface. The wound may evolve rapidly to reveal the actual extent of tissue injury, or may resolve without tissue loss. If necrotic tissue, subcutaneous tissue, granulation tissue, fascia, muscle, or other underlying structures are visible, this indicates a full thickness pressure injury (Unstageable, stage 3 or stage 4).

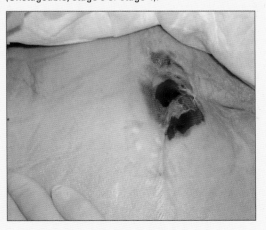

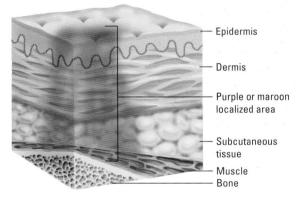

— Epidermis

— Dermis

— Purple or maroon localized area

— Subcutaneous tissue

— Muscle
— Bone

Stage 1

Stage 1 injuries are characterized by intact skin with a localized area of nonblanchable erythema, which may appear differently in darkly pigmented skin. Presence of blanchable erythema or changes in sensation, temperature, or firmness may precede visual changes. Color changes do not include purple or maroon discoloration; these may indicate deep tissue pressure injury.

To identify a stage 1 pressure injury, compare the suspected area to an adjacent area or to the same region on the other side of the body. Indications of stage 1 include differences in:

- skin temperature (warmth or coolness)
- tissue consistency (firm)
- sensation (pain).

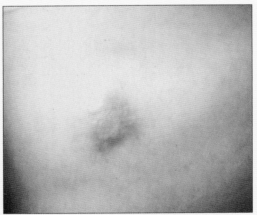

Stage 2

A stage 2 pressure injury is characterized by partial-thickness loss of the dermis The wound bed is viable, pink or red, moist, and may also present as an intact or ruptured serum-filled blister. Adipose (fat) is not visible, and deeper tissues are not visible. Granulation tissue, slough, and eschar are not present. These injuries commonly result from adverse microclimate and shear in the skin over the pelvis and shear in the heel. This is not the same as moisture-associated skin damage (MASD) such as incontinence-associated dermatitis (IAD), intertriginous dermatitis (ITD), medical adhesive–related skin injury (MARSI), or traumatic wounds (skin tears, burns, abrasions).

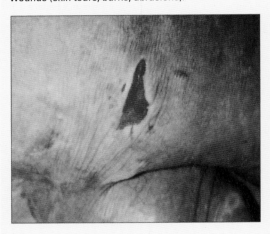

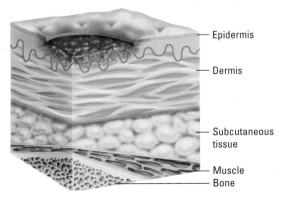

Stage 3

A stage 3 pressure injury is characterized by full-thickness loss of skin, in which adipose (fat) is visible in the ulcer and granulation tissue and epibole (rolled wound edges) are often present. Slough and/or eschar may be visible. The depth of tissue damage varies by anatomical location; areas of significant adiposity can develop deep wounds. Undermining and tunneling may occur. Fascia, muscle, tendon, ligament, cartilage, and/or bone are not exposed. If slough or eschar obscures the extent of tissue loss, this is an Unstageable Pressure Injury.

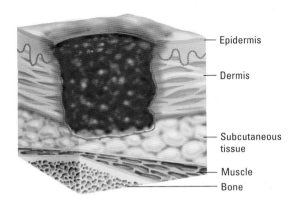

- Epidermis
- Dermis
- Subcutaneous tissue
- Muscle
- Bone

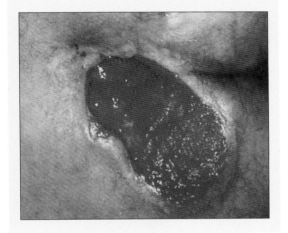

Stage 4

A stage 4 pressure injury is a full-thickness skin and tissue loss with exposed or directly palpable fascia, muscle, tendon, ligament, cartilage, or bone in the ulcer. Slough and/or eschar may be visible. Epibole (rolled edges), undermining, and/or tunneling often occur. Depth varies by anatomical location. If slough or eschar obscures the extent of tissue loss, this is an Unstageable Pressure Injury.

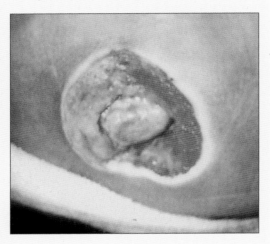

Unstageable

An unstageable injury is characterized by full-thickness skin and tissue loss in which the extent of tissue damage within the ulcer cannot be confirmed because it is obscured by slough or eschar. If slough or eschar is removed, a stage 3 or stage 4 pressure injury will be revealed. Stable eschar (i.e., dry, adherent, intact without erythema or fluctuance) on the heel or ischemic limb should not be softened or removed.

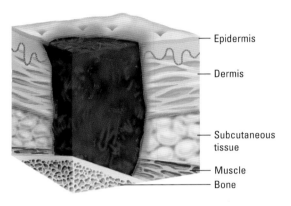

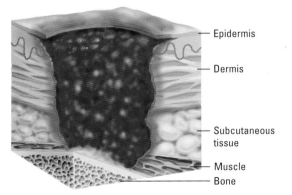

Medical device–related pressure injury

Medical device–related pressure injuries result from the use of devices designed and applied for diagnostic or therapeutic purposes and include catheters, braces, splints, casts, and respiratory devices such as endotracheal tubes and tracheostomy tubes. The resultant pressure injury generally conforms to the pattern or shape of the device. Stage this skin injury according to the staging system.

Mucosal membrane pressure injury

Mucosal membrane pressure injury is found on mucous membranes with a history of a medical device in use at the location of the injury. Due to the anatomy of the tissue, these ulcers cannot be staged.

Treatment

Treatment of pressure injuries includes nutritional assessment and support, management of tissue loads, wound care, and management of bacterial colonization and infection.

Management of pressure injury algorithm

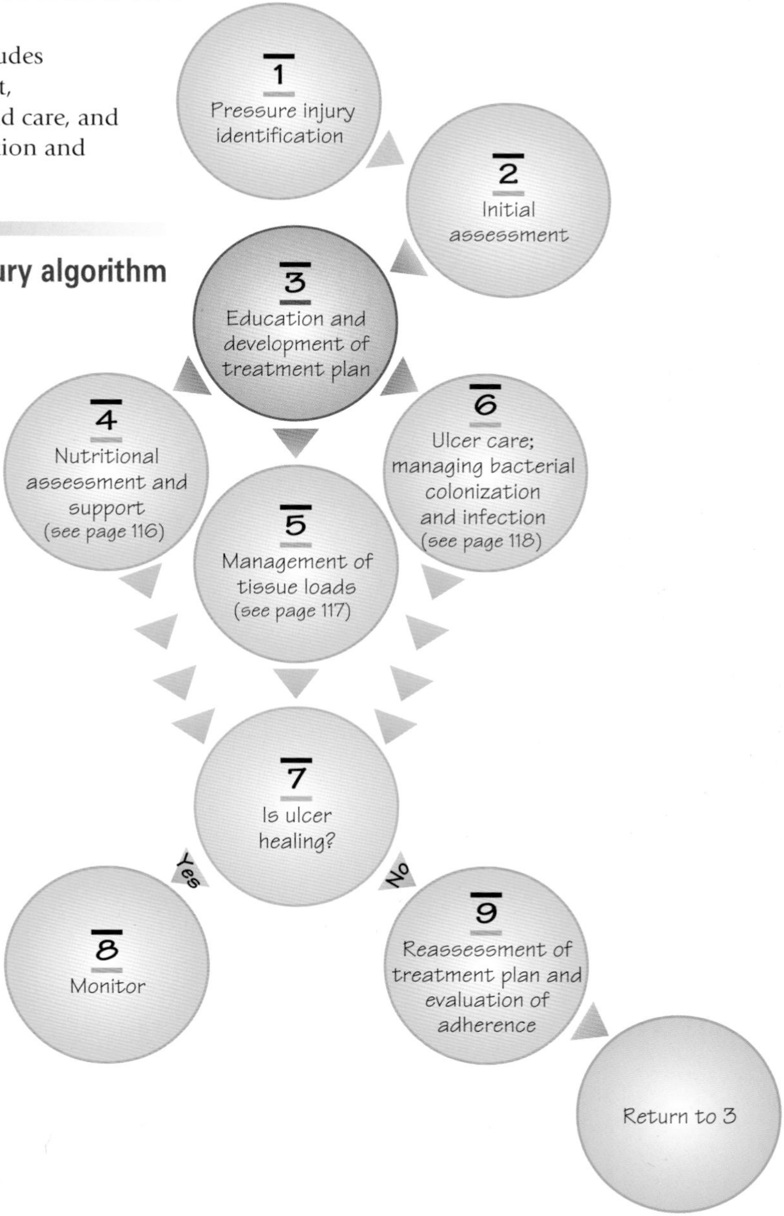

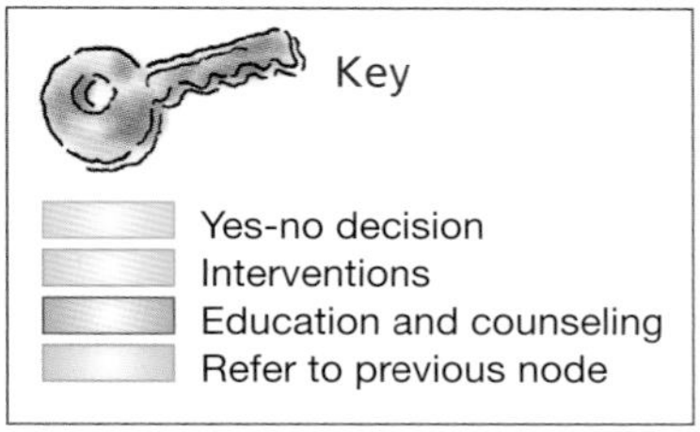

1 Pressure injury identification

2 Initial assessment

3 Education and development of treatment plan

4 Nutritional assessment and support (see page 116)

5 Management of tissue loads (see page 117)

6 Ulcer care; managing bacterial colonization and infection (see page 118)

7 Is ulcer healing?

8 Monitor

9 Reassessment of treatment plan and evaluation of adherence

Yes

No

Return to 3

Key

- Yes-no decision
- Interventions
- Education and counseling
- Refer to previous node

Nutritional assessment and support algorithm

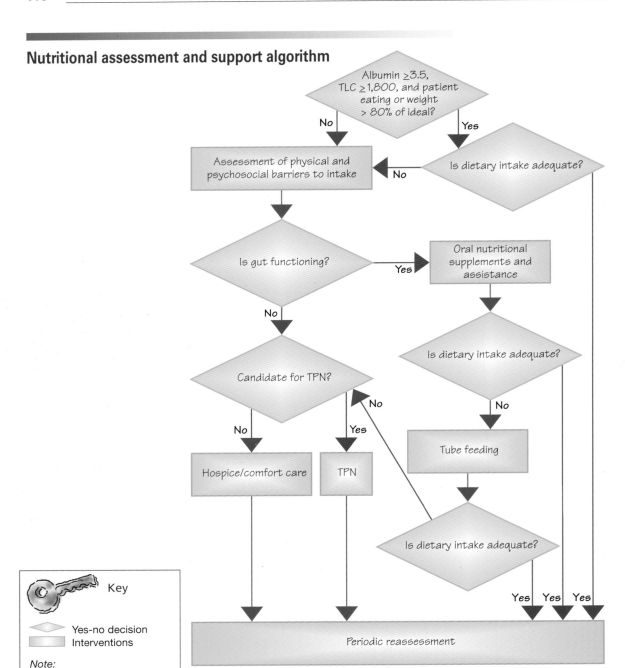

Management of tissue loads algorithm

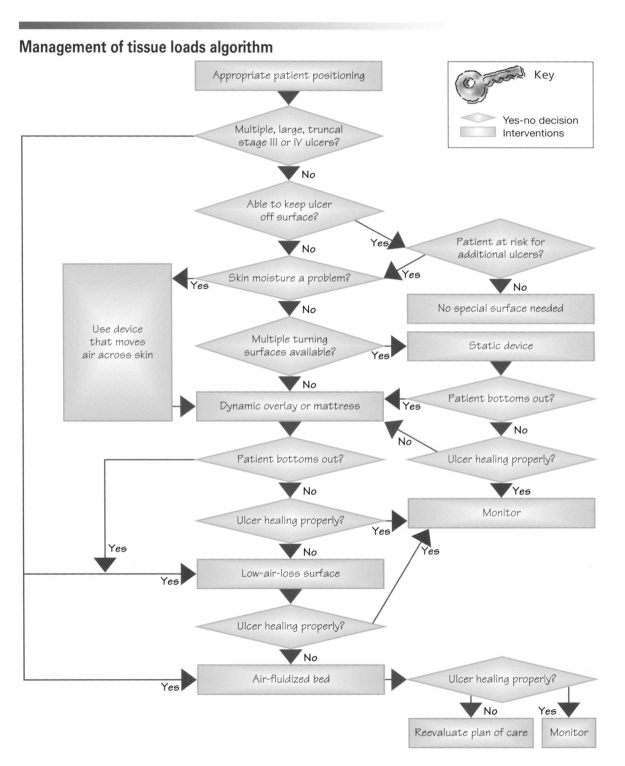

Management of bacterial colonization and infection algorithm

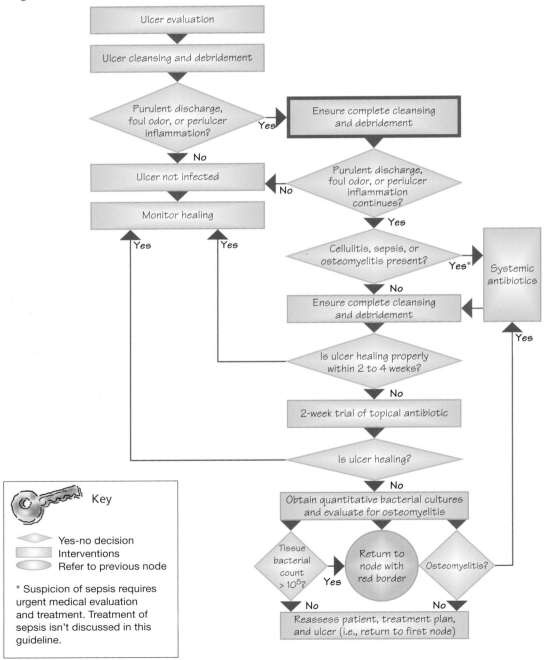

Ulcer evaluation

Ulcer cleansing and debridement

Purulent discharge, foul odor, or periulcer inflammation? — Yes → Ensure complete cleansing and debridement

No

Ulcer not infected

Monitor healing

Purulent discharge, foul odor, or periulcer inflammation continues? — No →

Yes

Cellulitis, sepsis, or osteomyelitis present? — Yes* → Systemic antibiotics

No

Ensure complete cleansing and debridement

Is ulcer healing properly within 2 to 4 weeks? — Yes

No

2-week trial of topical antibiotic

Is ulcer healing? — Yes

No

Obtain quantitative bacterial cultures and evaluate for osteomyelitis

Tissue bacterial count > 10^5? — Yes → Return to node with red border ← Osteomyelitis? — Yes

No — No

Reassess patient, treatment plan, and ulcer (i.e., return to first node)

Key

◇ Yes-no decision
▭ Interventions
⬭ Refer to previous node

* Suspicion of sepsis requires urgent medical evaluation and treatment. Treatment of sepsis isn't discussed in this guideline.

Pressure injury care

Assess for signs of pressure injury.

| Stage 1 | Stage 2, stage 3, or stage 4 |

Stage 1:
Wash gently with warm water or commercial skin cleanser, pat dry.

- Remove area from pressure sources.
- Assess other contributing factors to break in skin integrity.
  - Remediate other factors, if possible.

Stage 2, stage 3, or stage 4:
Irrigate wound bed with normal saline solution or ordered solution. Wash around wound bed with normal saline solution; pat dry.

- Assess color, odor, and amount of drainage on old dressing.
- Assess ulcer color, length, width, depth, and drainage.
- Assess for necrotic areas.
- Assess skin around wound. (Is it intact, macerated, inflamed, tunneled?)

Choose type of ulcer treatment. (Add moisture, remove moisture, use antibacterial, fill cavity, support autolysis of debris, totally occlude, partially occlude?)

Choose method of debridement (surgical or nonsurgical).

Choose care for periwound skin. (Keep dry, use protective barrier, avoid adhesives?)

Choose a dressing. (Primary with separate secondary, combination?) Initiate and maintain pressure preventive measures and remediation of any other contributing factors, if possible.

Regularly reassess effectiveness of interventions.

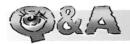

Matchmaker

Match the six illustrations of pressure injuries with their correct stage.

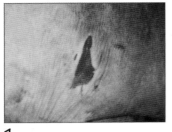

1. _____

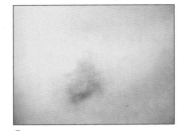

2. _____

A. Stage 1

B. Stage 2

C. Stage 3

D. Stage 4

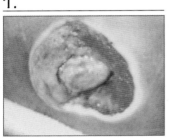

3. _____

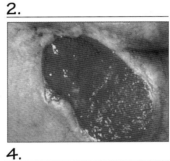

4. _____

Able to label?

Label the pressure points susceptible to ulcer formation in the illustration.

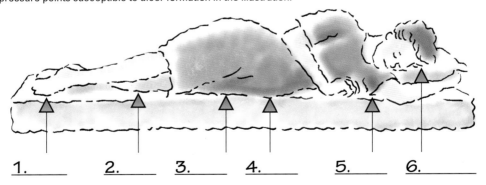

1. _____ 2. _____ 3. _____ 4. _____ 5. _____ 6. _____

Suggested References

Braden, B., & Bergstrom, N. (1988). Braden scale for predicting pressure ulcer risk. Retrieved from http://www.bradenscale.com/images/bradenscale.pdf

Coleman, S., Gorecki, C., Nelson, E. A., Closs, J., Deloor, T., Halfens, R., ..., Nixon, J. (2013). Patient risk factors for pressure ulcer development: Systematic review. *International Journal of Nursing Studies, 50*(7), 974–1003.

Edsberg, L., Black, J., Goldberg, M., McNichol, L., Moore, L., & Sieggreen, M. (2016). Revised national pressure injury advisory panel pressure ulcer staging system: Revised pressure injury staging system. *Journal of Wound, Ostomy, and Continence Nursing, 43*(6), 585–597.

Kelechi, T., Arndt, J., & Dove, A. (2013). Review of pressure ulcer risk assessment scales. *Journal of Wound, Ostomy, and Continence Nursing, 40*(3), 232–236.

McNichol, L., Watts, C., Mackey, D., Beitz, J., & Gray, M. (2015). Identifying the right surface for the right patient at the right time: Generation and content validation of an algorithm for support surface selection. *Journal of Wound, Ostomy, and Continence Nursing, 42*(1), 19–37.

NPUAP. (2016). NPUAP pressure injury stages. Retrieved from http://www.npuap.org/resources/educational-and-clinical-resources/npuap-pressure-injury-stages/

Nestle. (2010). Algorithm for treatment of pressure ulcers: Nutrition guidelines. Retrieved from http:///www.nestle-nutrition.com/nirf/cm2/upload/C2F33D34-9316-4155-9F0F-58FDD9E638D9/Treatment-decision-tree-pressure-ulcers-final-8-5-10.pdf

National Pressure Ulcer Advisory Panel, European Pressure Ulcer Advisory Panel and Pan Pacific Pressure Injury Alliance. (2014). In E. Haesler (Ed.), *Prevention and treatment of pressure ulcers: Quick reference guide.* Osborne Park, Australia: Cambridge Media.

Vascular ulcers

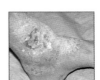

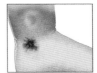

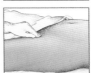

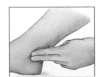

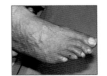

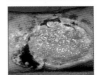

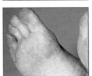

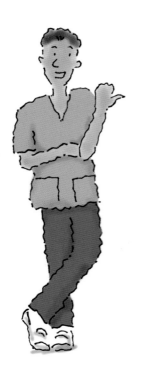

Vascular system

The body's vascular system consists of:
- veins (carry blood toward the heart)
- arteries (carry blood away from the heart)
- lymphatic system (a separate circulatory system that collects waste products and delivers them to the venous system).

Veins

Veins carry deoxygenated blood back to the heart for reoxygenation.

A close look at a vein

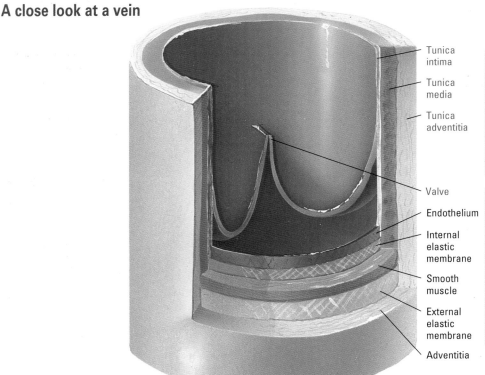

Tunica intima

Tunica media

Tunica adventitia

Valve

Endothelium

Internal elastic membrane

Smooth muscle

External elastic membrane

Adventitia

Vein walls have three layers. Compared to arteries of the same size, veins have thinner walls and wider diameters.

Veins have a unique system of cup-shaped valves that open toward the heart. The valves function to keep blood flowing in one direction—toward the heart.

Major lower limb veins

The illustration below shows the major veins in this part of the body.

Types of veins

The lower portion of the body contains three major types of veins and smaller vessels known as venules. Venules are very small veins whose purpose is to collect blood from the small capillaries in the arterial system.

Superficial veins

Superficial veins lie just beneath the skin; they drain through perforator veins into deep veins.

Perforator veins

Perforator veins connect superficial to deep veins.

Deep veins

Deep veins receive venous blood from perforator veins and return it to the heart.

He's really a superficial vein. He just thinks if he reads enough literature, people will start to think he's deep.

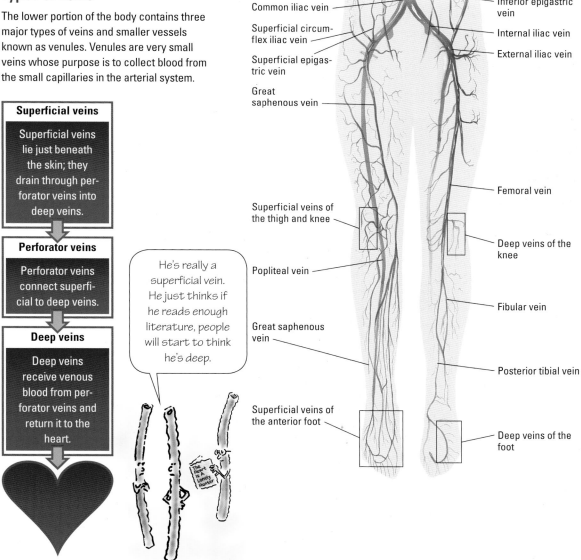

Abdominal vena cava

Common iliac vein

Superficial circumflex iliac vein

Superficial epigastric vein

Great saphenous vein

Inferior epigastric vein

Internal iliac vein

External iliac vein

Femoral vein

Superficial veins of the thigh and knee

Deep veins of the knee

Popliteal vein

Fibular vein

Great saphenous vein

Posterior tibial vein

Superficial veins of the anterior foot

Deep veins of the foot

Arteries

Arteries carry blood from the heart to every functioning cell in the body. The lower portion of the body receives its arterial flow through the abdominal aorta and the major arteries branching from it.

A close look at an artery

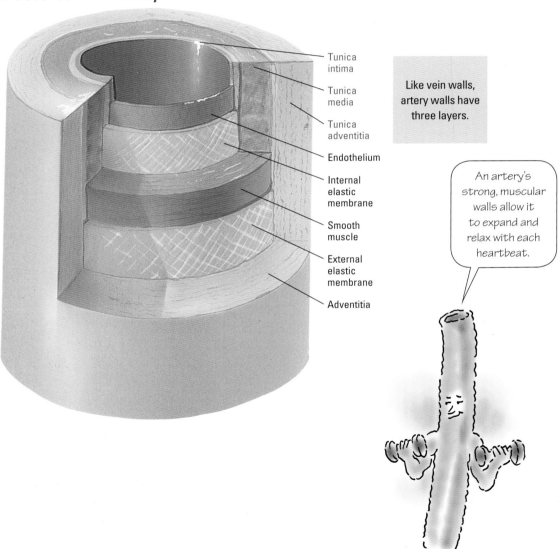

Tunica intima

Tunica media

Tunica adventitia

Endothelium

Internal elastic membrane

Smooth muscle

External elastic membrane

Adventitia

Like vein walls, artery walls have three layers.

An artery's strong, muscular walls allow it to expand and relax with each heartbeat.

Major lower limb arteries

This illustration identifies the major arteries in the lower portion of the body. Capillaries are the smallest of the blood vessels and make up the body's microcirculation. They connect arterioles and venules and facilitate movement of water, oxygen, carbon dioxide, and other substances between the tissues and blood around them.

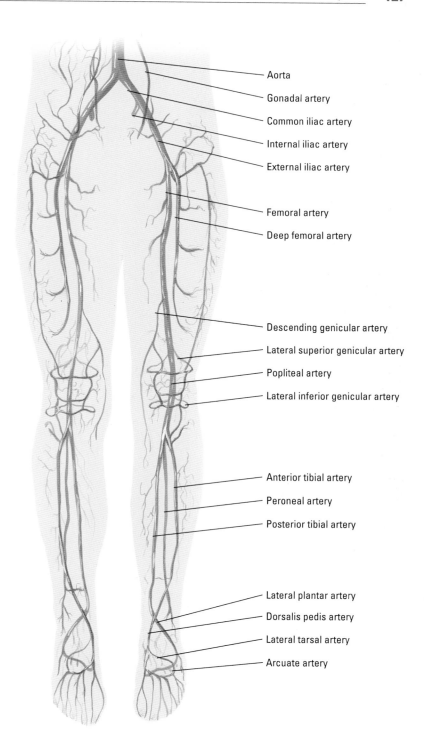

- Aorta
- Gonadal artery
- Common iliac artery
- Internal iliac artery
- External iliac artery
- Femoral artery
- Deep femoral artery
- Descending genicular artery
- Lateral superior genicular artery
- Popliteal artery
- Lateral inferior genicular artery
- Anterior tibial artery
- Peroneal artery
- Posterior tibial artery
- Lateral plantar artery
- Dorsalis pedis artery
- Lateral tarsal artery
- Arcuate artery

Assessing lower extremity pulses

Assessing pulses is an effective way to evaluate arterial blood flow to the lower extremities. These illustrations show where to position your fingers when palpating for pulses of the lower extremities. Use your index and middle fingers to apply pressure.

Femoral pulse

Press firmly at a point inferior to the inguinal ligament. For obese patients, palpate in the groin crease, halfway between the pubic bone and hip bone.

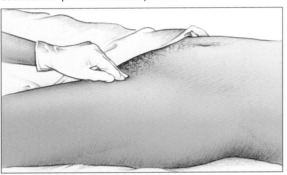

Popliteal pulse

Press firmly in the popliteal fossa at the back of the knee.

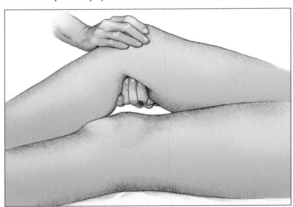

Posterior tibial pulse

Apply pressure behind and slightly below the medial malleolus.

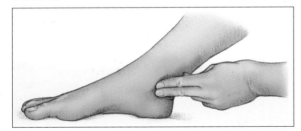

Dorsalis pedis pulse

Place your fingers on the medial dorsum of the foot while the patient points his toes down. The pulse is difficult to palpate here and may seem absent in healthy patients. Sometimes, it helps to dorsiflex the foot to "pop up" the artery that lies between the first and second metatarsal bones.

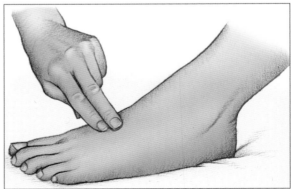

Using a Doppler to assess blood flow

In Doppler ultrasonography, high-frequency sound waves are used to assess blood flow. A handheld transducer, or probe, directs the sound waves into a vessel, where they strike moving red blood cells (RBCs). The frequency of the sound waves changes in proportion to the velocity of the RBCs. Doppler ultrasonography can be used to assess both arterial and venous blood flow.

Assessing arterial blood flow

- Apply a small amount of transmission gel to the ultrasound probe.
- Position the probe on the skin directly over the selected artery.
- Turn the instrument on and set the volume to the lowest setting.
- To obtain the best signal, tilt the probe at a 45-degree angle from the artery, making sure that the gel is between the skin and the probe.
- Slowly move the probe in a circular motion to locate the center of the artery. Avoid pressing the probe too heavily on the artery to avoid compressing it.
- Listen for a triphasic, biphasic, or monophasic sound, which occurs when the Doppler signal isolates an artery.
- Count the signal for 60 seconds to determine the pulse rate.

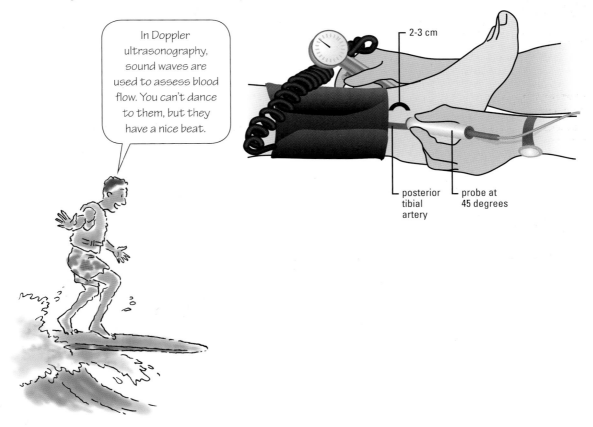

Measuring ankle-brachial index

The ankle-brachial index (ABI) is a value derived from blood pressure measurements, which shows the progress or improvement of arterial disease. Each value in the index is a ratio of blood pressure measurement in the affected limb to the highest systolic pressure in the brachial arteries.

Steps
- Place the patient in a supine position with the legs at heart level.
- Measure and record both brachial blood pressures.
- Wrap the blood pressure cuff around one ankle, just above the malleolus, with the cuff bladder centered over the posterior tibial artery.
- Apply ultrasound transmission gel to a Doppler transducer.
- Hold the Doppler transducer over the dorsalis pedis artery at a 45-degree angle.
- Inflate the blood pressure cuff until the Doppler signal disappears.
- Slowly deflate the cuff until the Doppler signal returns. Record this pressure as the dorsalis pedis pressure.
- Repeat this same procedure over the posterior tibial artery. Record this pressure as the posterior tibial pressure.
- Calculate the ABI by dividing the highest ankle pressure by the highest brachial systolic pressure.
- Repeat the process on the contralateral limb.

Interpretation of results
- ABI > 0.9 = Normal
- ABI 0.71 to 0.9 = Mild arterial insufficiency
- ABI 0.41 to 0.7 = Moderate arterial insufficiency
- ABI 0 to 0.40 = Severe arterial insufficiency

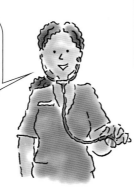

The ABI may not be accurate in patients with diabetes or arterial medial calcinosis.

Ankle-brachial index (ABI) worksheet

Patient Name _____

Date _____ Patient number _____

Right Arm
Systolic Pressure:
_____

Left Arm
Systolic Pressure:
_____

Right Ankle
Systolic Pressure:

Left Ankle
Systolic Pressure:

Posterior tibial (PT) _____   _____ Posterior tibial (PT)
Dorsal pedis (DP) _____   _____ Dorsal pedis (DP)

Right ABI

$$\frac{\text{Higher Right Ankle Pressure}}{\text{Higher Arm Pressure}} = \frac{\text{mm Hg}}{\text{mm Hg}} = \underline{\quad}$$

Left ABI

$$\frac{\text{Higher Right Ankle Pressure}}{\text{Higher Arm Pressure}} = \frac{\text{mm Hg}}{\text{mm Hg}} = \underline{\quad}$$

Example

$$\frac{\text{Higher Ankle Pressure}}{\text{Higher Brachial Pressure}} = \frac{\text{mm Hg}}{\text{mm Hg}} \quad \underline{\quad}$$

Lymphatic system

The lymphatic system is a vascular network that drains lymph (a protein-rich fluid similar to plasma) from body tissues and intravascular compartments and returns it to the venous system.

Lymphatic system and drainage route

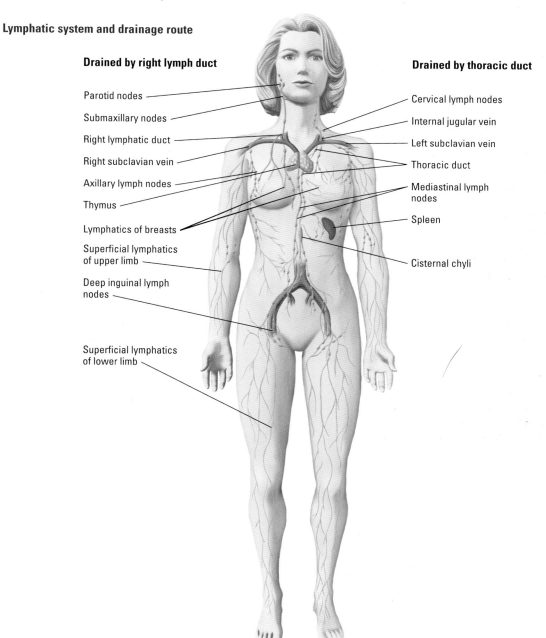

Drained by right lymph duct

Parotid nodes

Submaxillary nodes

Right lymphatic duct

Right subclavian vein

Axillary lymph nodes

Thymus

Lymphatics of breasts

Superficial lymphatics of upper limb

Deep inguinal lymph nodes

Superficial lymphatics of lower limb

Drained by thoracic duct

Cervical lymph nodes

Internal jugular vein

Left subclavian vein

Thoracic duct

Mediastinal lymph nodes

Spleen

Cisternal chyli

The lymphatic system begins peripherally, with lymph capillaries that absorb fluid. The capillaries proceed centrally to thin vascular vessels. These vessels empty into collecting ducts, which empty into major veins at the base of the neck.

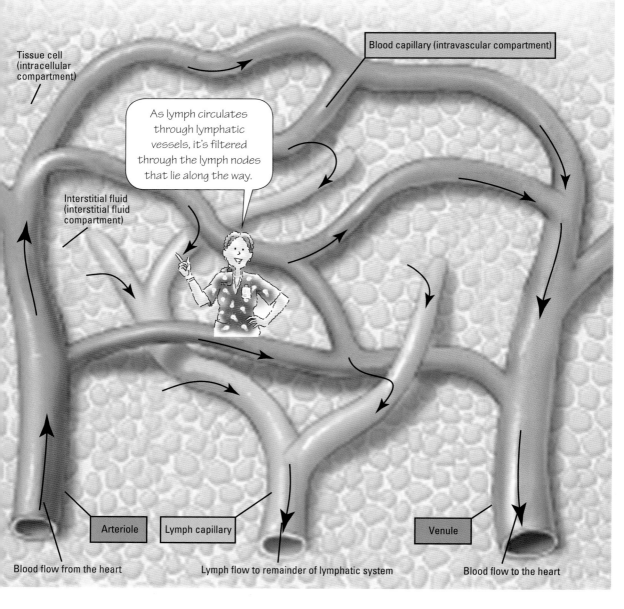

Vascular disorders

Venous

Venous disorders are the most common type of vascular conditions and encompass venous insufficiency, venous disease, and other conditions such as venous thromboembolism. The primary cause of venous insufficiency is hypertension in the venous system or obstructions from blood clots, whereas venous disease is a progressive disorder that leads to damaged veins and at worst, ulceration.

When leg veins fail to propel a sufficient supply of blood back to the heart, blood begins to pool in the legs (venous insufficiency). Causes of venous insufficiency include:

- **incompetent valves**—most common cause; can result when a blood clot disrupts valve function or when a vein distends (venous hypertension) to the point that the valve no longer closes completely
- **inadequate calf muscle function**
- **poor range of motion of the ankle**
- **damaged perforator veins**

Major risk factors for venous insufficiency include:

- older age
- female sex
- obesity
- prolonged sitting or standing
- family history
- lower leg trauma
- venous thromboembolism (deep vein thrombosis)
- pregnancy

Signs of venous insufficiency are progressive and classified as follows:
• Edema is one of the first signs and can pitting or nonpitting.
• Telangiectasia—the superficial veins just below the skin's surface become dilated, producing a weblike appearance of the skin, sometimes referred to as spider veins.
• Hyperpigmentation in calves and around the gaiter area (between malleoli and calves) due to buildup of hemosiderin as a result from breakdown of red blood cells that have leaked into tissue, sometimes referred to as brown staining.
• Atrophie blanche appears as round spots of ivory white plaque in skin, usually surrounded by hyperpigmentation.
• Lipodermatosclerosis is a hardening condition of the skin caused by inflammation of the fat that can cause a constriction around the lower leg that makes the legs giving the appearance of an upside down champagne bottle.
• Venous eczema is characterized by red, flaky sometimes raised areas referred to as stasis dermatitis.
• Venous ulceration is the most severe consequence of venous disease, which results in tissue loss.

Symptoms of venous insufficiency include:

Many patients report dull, aching pain, or heaviness that is relieved by elevation of the leg. Itching, throbbing, burning, and muscle cramps during walking or exercising (venous claudication) are other commonly reported symptoms. Feelings of irritability and fatigue are prevalent.

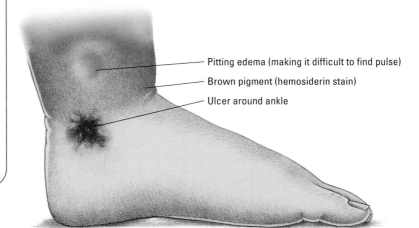

Pitting edema (making it difficult to find pulse)
Brown pigment (hemosiderin stain)
Ulcer around ankle

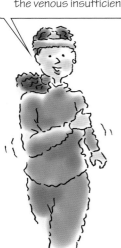

Physical activity is crucial to adequate venous return. Leg muscle paralysis or prolonged inactivity such as bed rest during hospitalization can drastically hinder the amount of blood returning to the heart. It then pools in the legs, causing swelling, and putting patients at risk for blood clots. Patients will have some types of venous embolism prevention in place in the hospital such as stockings or pumps. When discharged, they will require higher compression to manage the venous insufficiency.

Arterial

Understanding atherosclerosis

Arterial insufficiency is most commonly associated with artherosclerosis. In atherosclerosis, fatty, fibrous plaques progressively narrow the arterial lumen. This reduces blood flow and leads to tissue ischemia. The illustrations below show the progression of atherosclerosis.

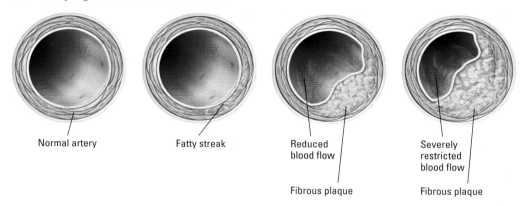

Normal artery   Fatty streak   Reduced blood flow   Severely restricted blood flow

Fibrous plaque   Fibrous plaque

Risk factors for atherosclerosis
- Advanced age
- Smoking
- Obesity
- Hyperlipidemia
- Diabetes mellitus
- Hypertension
- Sedentary lifestyle

Other causes of arterial insufficiency include arterial stenosis (narrowing) or obstruction (from thrombosis, emboli, vasculitis, or Raynaud's phenomenon).

Signs and symptoms of arterial insufficiency

- Dependent rubor is a change in color of the skin to a deep bluish-red when the patient places the foot in a dependent position to ischemic changes due to ischemia.
- Very slender lower extremity from lack of blood flow to muscle.
- Thin, pale brittle or crumbly yellow nails. Nails may be thickened as a result of arterial insufficiency or from fungal infection.
- Claudication is when pain is manifested distal to a narrowed artery brought on by exercise and relieved by rest. Rest pain often signals severe disease and occurs in the foot when the patient is asleep, relieved by lowering extremity over the side of the bed.

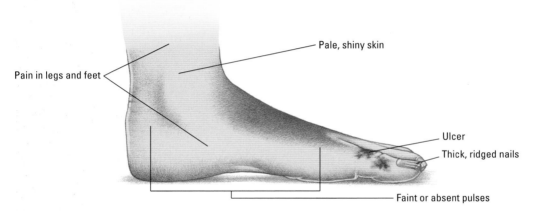

Pain in legs and feet

Pale, shiny skin

Ulcer

Thick, ridged nails

Faint or absent pulses

Identifying dependent rubor

Dependent rubor is a sign of chronic arterial insufficiency. To elicit this sign during a physical examination:

• Elevate the foot with the ulcer to a 30-degree angle. If the foot is ischemic, the skin will pale.

• Ask the patient to lower the foot into a dependent position. Ischemic skin becomes deep red as the tissue fills with blood. This dramatic color change—called *dependent rubor*—signifies severe tissue ischemia.

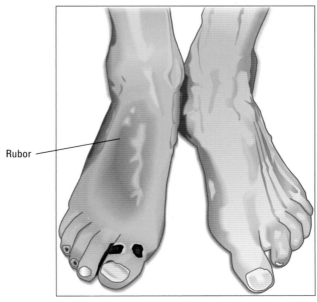

Rubor

Lymphedema

Understanding lymphedema

Lymphedema occurs when an obstruction in the lymphatic system causes lymphatic fluid to build up in the interstitial spaces of body tissues. In the legs, the steady seepage of fluid into interstitial tissues can result in massive edema, as shown here.

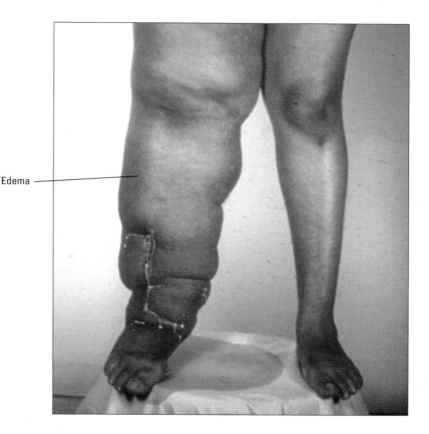

Edema

Signs of lymphedema

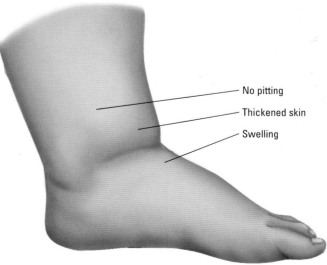

No pitting

Thickened skin

Swelling

Vascular ulcers

Disorders of the venous, arterial, and lymphatic systems can cause wounds, called *vascular ulcers,* to develop. Vascular ulcers occur most commonly on the lower extremities. Chronic ulcers are defined as those that fail to heal or show any signs of healing after 4 weeks.

Types of vascular ulcers

Type of ulcer	Typical location	Clinical findings
Venous	• Anywhere from ankle to midcalf • Most common on medial aspect of ankle above the malleolus	• Irregular shape that can be quite large • Can drain heavily but can also become dry, crusted, or moist, slightly macerated borders • Shallow wound base covered with beefy red granulation tissue, yellow film, or gray necrotic tissue (black necrotic tissue rarely present except in acute injury)
Arterial	• Tips of toes, corners of nail beds on toes, over bony prominences, and between toes	• Pale or mottled wound, generally small in size that can look "punched out" • Well-demarcated wound edges • Dry wound base with no granulation tissue (due to impaired blood flow to tissue) • Presence of necrotic tissue (commonly) or hard, dark dry leatherly eschar • Surrounding skin that feels cooler than normal on palpation
Lymphatic	• Arms and legs, most commonly ankle area; these ulcers are rare	• Shallow ulcer bed that may be oozing, moist, or blistered • Firm, fibrotic surrounding skin that's thickened by edema • Cellulitis (possibly)

Between 70% and 90% of all leg ulcers are venous ulcers and most commonly occur on the lower extremities between the malleoli and calves, also known as the gaiter area.

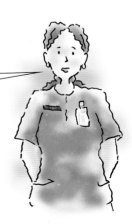

A closer look at venous ulcers

Venous ulcers most commonly occur above the medial malleolus. These ulcers have irregular borders and typically appear moist.

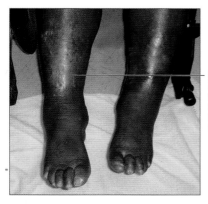

Swelling of the lower legs with brown discoloration and small ulcers characterize venous insufficiency.

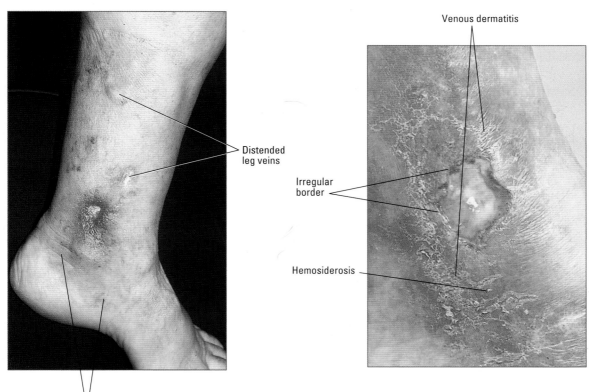

Venous dermatitis

Distended leg veins

Irregular border

Hemosiderosis

Telangiectasis

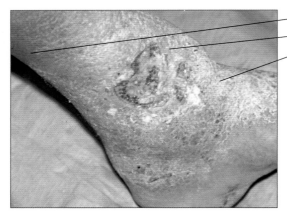

- Hemosiderosis
- Lipodermatosclerosis
- Venous dermatitis

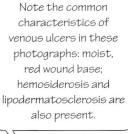

Note the common characteristics of venous ulcers in these photographs: moist, red wound base; hemosiderosis and lipodermatosclerosis are also present.

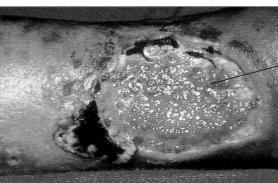

- Moist, beefy red wound base

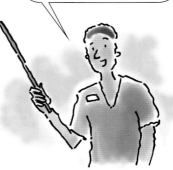

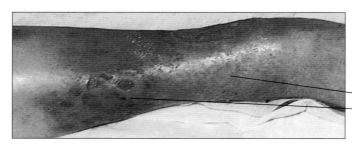

- Lipodermatosclerosis
- Hemosiderosis

Care considerations

For heavily draining ulcers, the goal is to absorb the drainage and prevent maceration of the surrounding skin. If pain is present, dressings can be selected to reduce discomfort. Using compression bandages such as multilayer wraps is the hallmark of treatment to reduce edema.

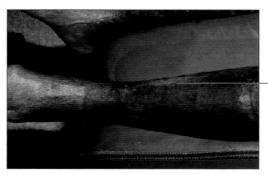

- Hard thickened lipodermatosclerotic skin is easily traumatized and can lead to ulcers.

Arterial ulcers

Also called *ischemic ulcers,* arterial ulcers result from tissue ischemia caused by insufficient blood flow through an artery (arterial insufficiency). Arterial ulcers most commonly occur in the area around the toes.

Development of an arterial ulcer

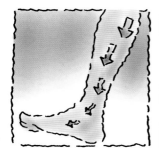 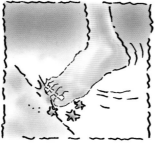 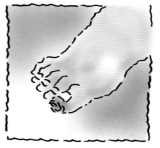

1 Arterial flow is diminished.

2 Trauma occurs to an area with arterial insufficiency.

3 Reduced blood flow impairs healing, resulting in a chronic wound, meaning, healing will not take place or takes place over many weeks to months.

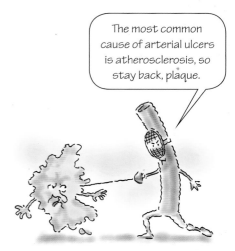

The most common cause of arterial ulcers is atherosclerosis, so stay back, plaque.

A closer look at arterial ulcers

Arterial ulcers usually have well-demarcated edges. Because of decreased blood flow, the base of the ulcer is typically pale and dry and granulation tissue may be absent. On examination, you may notice an area of wet necrosis or a dry scab. The skin surrounding the ulcer will feel cooler than normal.

Common sites of arterial ulcers include the tips of the toes, the corners of nail beds on the toes, over bony prominences, and between toes.

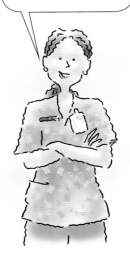

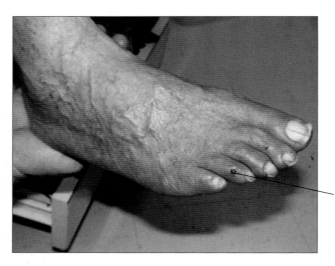

Arterial toe ulcer

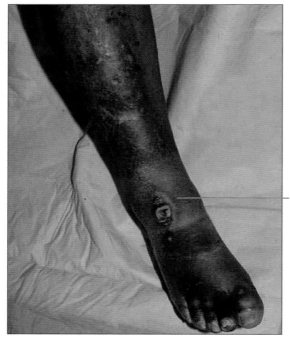

Ulcers on lower leg and 2nd toe resulting from critical limb ischema.

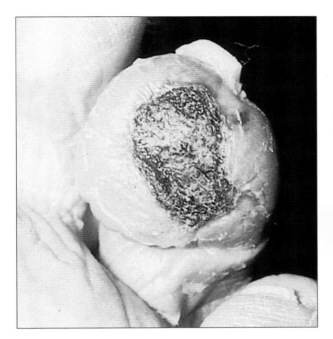

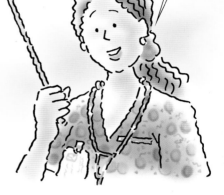

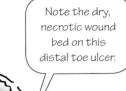

Care considerations

The goal of nursing care is to protect the affected skin by covering the wound with nonadherent dressings. Often the patient will need revascularization procedures to enhance blood flow. Patients should be encouraged to walk and exercise and stop smoking. Many walking and smoking cessation programs are readily available.

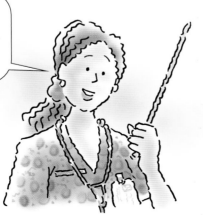

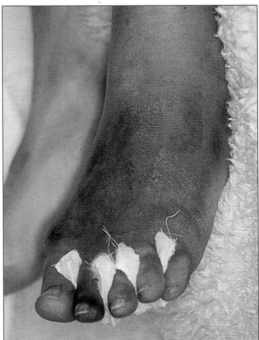

Lymphatic ulcers

Lymphatic ulcers result when a part of the body afflicted with lymphedema suffers an injury. Here are some predisposing factors for ulcer formation:

- **Pressure on capillaries**—The skin and underlying tissue in areas with lymphedema become firm and fibrotic over time. This thickened tissue presses on capillaries, occluding blood flow and leaving the area vulnerable to ulcer formation. Because of the poor circulation, these ulcers are extremely difficult to treat.
- **Skin folds from massive swelling**—Skin folds can trap moisture, leading to tissue maceration and ulcer formation.
- **Traumatic injury or pressure**—Pressure or injury in an area with lymphedema commonly leads to an ulcer.

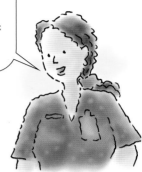

Lymphatic ulcers commonly occur in the ankle area, but they can develop at any site of traumatic injury in an area with lymphedema.

A closer look at lymphatic ulcers

Lymphatic ulcers are typically shallow and may be oozing, moist, or blistered. The surrounding skin is usually firm, fibrotic, and thickened by edema. Cellulitis (tissue inflammation) may also be present. Dry, warty spots called *papillomatoses* may develop.

Care considerations

Use of an absorbent dressing is often required because these ulcers generally have high drainage until the edema is controlled. It is important to keep the skin around the ulcers clean, dry, and moisturized. If there is excessive drainage from the ulcer, a moisture barrier will be needed.

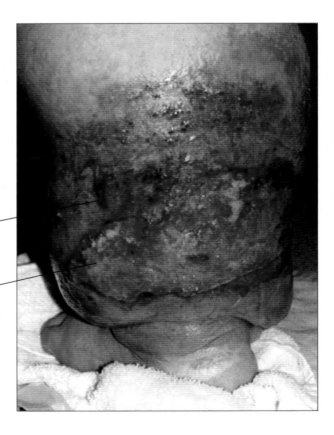

Papillomatosis —

Shallow, moist lymphatic ulcer —

Treatment

Effective treatment of a vascular ulcer involves caring for the wound as well as managing the underlying vascular disease. The goals and treatment recommendations vary depending on the type of ulcer.

Type of ulcer	Treatment goals	Therapies and procedures	Wound care
Venous	• Control edema • Manage underlying venous disease • Provide appropriate wound care	• Limb elevation to allow gravity to drain fluid from the limb • Compression bandages, layered compression bandages, elastic bandages, compression pumps, compression stockings, or graduated compression support hosiery to reduce edema • Bandaging and wrapping (paste wrap such as Unna's boot) may be used to provide compression, protection, and a moist environment for healing	• Apply dressings to promote moist wound healing, growth of granulation tissue, and reepithelialization. • Apply growth factors to the wound bed, as ordered, to improve healing rate. • Consider advanced wound healing technologies such as cellular tissue products (CTPS) for a venous ulcer that fails to heal within 4 weeks of treatment.
Arterial	• Reestablish arterial flow • Provide appropriate wound care and wound protection	• Arterial bypass to restore arterial flow • Angioplasty (with possible stent insertion) to treat arterial stenosis	• Keep the wound dry and protected from pressure or trauma. • As ordered, apply an antiseptic or antimicrobial agent and then place small gauze pads between the toes. Change the pads daily to keep toe ulcers dry. • Never soak arterial ulcers. • If revascularization succeeds, change the type of dressing to keep moist tissue moist and dry tissue dry.
Lymphatic	• Reduce edema • Prevent infection • Provide appropriate wound care	• Limb elevation and compression pump therapy to reduce edema • Comprehensive decongestive therapy (a form of massage) to reduce edema and improve circulation	• Follow guidelines for venous ulcer care. • Choose dressings that can manage large fluid loads while protecting the surrounding skin, such as foams and other absorbent dressings. • Negative pressure wound therapy may be a good alternative to dressings for copious fluid leakage.

Treatment of venous ulcers algorithm

Establish etiology.
Review patient history and
wound management.
Perform leg examination.

Arterial complications?

Yes → Vascular consult

No → **Debridement?**

Yes →

Necrotic tissue
Removal of necrotic tissue:
- Autolytic debridement
- Sharp debridement
- Enzymatic debridement

No →

Infection?

Yes →

Fibrotic tissue
Small amounts: Leave intact.
Moderate to large amounts:
- Autolytic debridement
- Sharp debridement
- Enzymatic debridement

Yes →

Localized
Treatment:
Dressing management
Use an antimicrobial
dressing based on
amount of drainage
from hydrdogel,
alginate/hydrofber,
or foam category
Cadexomer iodine
gel or pads

No →

Dressing management based on amount of wound drainage
- Alginate/hydrofiber dressings
- Hydrogel dressings
- Foam dressings
- Cellular tissue products
- Drugs (fibrinolytic agents or pentoxifylline [Trental])

Yes →

Systemic
Treatment:
- Outpatient oral or I.V. antibiotics
- In patient I.V. antibiotics
- No occlusive management modalities

Compression management?

Yes →
- Stockings
- Inelastic compression system (Unna's boot)
- Elastic compression system (multilayer sustained graduated compression system)
- Pumps

Reevaluation

No →
- Infection   ■ Arterial disease
- Weeping dermatitis ■ Heart failure

→ Consult physician

→ Choose appropriate management modalities

How to wrap Unna's boot and similar compression bandages

- Clean the patient's skin thoroughly.
- Flex the patient's knee.
- With the foot positioned at a right angle to the leg, wrap the medicated gauze bandage firmly—not tightly—around the patient's foot. Make sure the dressing covers the heel.
- Continue wrapping upward, overlapping the layers by 50% with each turn. Make sure that the layering circles the leg at an angle to avoid compromising the circulation. Smooth the boot with your free hand as you go, as shown below.

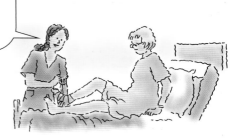

A treatment for venous ulcers involves applying an inelastic compression system called Unna's boot.

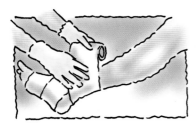

- Stop wrapping about 1" (2.5 cm) below the knee, as shown below. If constriction develops as the dressing hardens, make a 2" (5.1-cm) slit in the boot just below the knee.

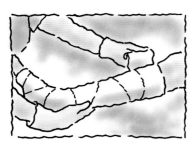

- If drainage is excessive, wrap a roller gauze dressing over the boot.
- Finally, wrap the boot with an elastic bandage in a figure-of-8 pattern, as shown below.

Take note

Documenting compression bandage application

1/2/18	1030	Compression wrap applied to pt's right leg at 0930. Assessment revealed a 3cm length, 1.5cm width, 0.2cm depth venous ulcer, located 5cm above right medial malleolus. Wound bed appears moist and beefy red. Mild serous drainage noted on the dressing that was removed; no odor noted. Surrounding skin dry and scaly indicative of slight venous eczema, but intact. Right lower extremity dorsalis pedis and posterior tibial pulses easily palpable. Wound cleaned with NSS and patted dry thoroughly. A moisture barrier ointment was applied to periwound skin and a thin, nonadherent foam dressing covered the wound. A new multilayer compression bandage was applied, starting at the base of the toes wrapped to just below the knee. Toes on right foot presently appear pink with immediate capillary refill, no edema, normal sensation. Pt. tolerated procedure well. The patient was instructed to keep the leg elevated during the day, to drink plenty of fluids and maintain proper nutrition.

———— Isa Rapp, R.N.

Treatment of arterial ulcers algorithm

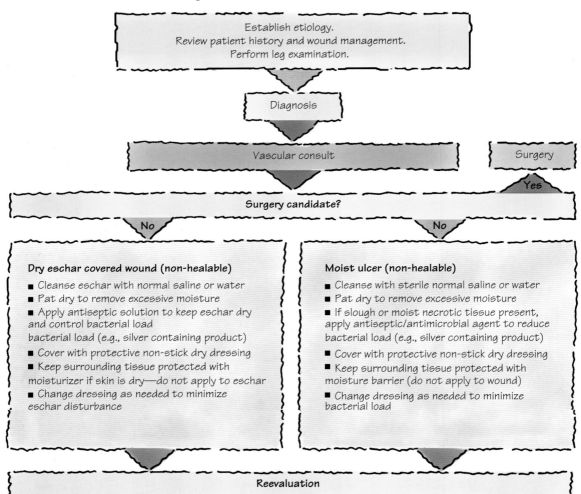

Establish etiology.
Review patient history and wound management.
Perform leg examination.

Diagnosis

Vascular consult

Surgery

Surgery candidate?

Yes

No

No

Dry eschar covered wound (non-healable)

- Cleanse eschar with normal saline or water
- Pat dry to remove excessive moisture
- Apply antiseptic solution to keep eschar dry and control bacterial load bacterial load (e.g., silver containing product)
- Cover with protective non-stick dry dressing
- Keep surrounding tissue protected with moisturizer if skin is dry—do not apply to eschar
- Change dressing as needed to minimize eschar disturbance

Moist ulcer (non-healable)

- Cleanse with sterile normal saline or water
- Pat dry to remove excessive moisture
- If slough or moist necrotic tissue present, apply antiseptic/antimicrobial agent to reduce bacterial load (e.g., silver containing product)
- Cover with protective non-stick dry dressing
- Keep surrounding tissue protected with moisture barrier (do not apply to wound)
- Change dressing as needed to minimize bacterial load

Reevaluation

* Do not debride arterial ulcers. The hard covering (eschar) should not be disturbed; it should be protected. Be careful not to disturb the already compromised arteries.

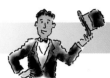

Dressings for vascular ulcers

Dressing	Indications and contraindications		
	Venous ulcers	*Arterial ulcers*	*Lymphatic ulcers*
Alginate/ hydrofiber	• Use to manage copious drainage.	• Use to manage copious drainage.	• Use to manage copious drainage.
Foam	• Use to protect the ulcer. • Use for absorption underneath a compression dressing.	• Use to protect the ulcer. • Use with dry gangrene. • Use for a moist, revascularized ulcer.	• Use to protect the ulcer. • Use to absorb drainage.
Hydrocolloid	• Use to promote granulation. • Use to manage pain. • Don't use when copious drainage is present.	• Use for autolytic debridement. • Use for primary dressing after revascularization. • Don't use on ischemic tissue. • Don't use when infection or cellulitis is present.	• Use to protect the skin. • Use to promote epithelialization. • Don't use when copious drainage is present. • Don't use when cellulitis is present.
Hydrogel	• Don't use when copious drainage is present.	• Use to maintain a moist wound bed. • Use for autolytic debridement.	• Use to manage pain. • Use for autolytic debridement.
Transparent film	• Use isn't indicated.	• Use only after the ulcer has almost completely healed.	• Use to protect fragile skin.

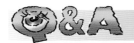

Matchmaker

Match the three types of ulcers shown here with their names.

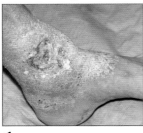

1. _____

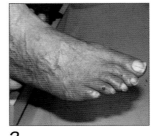

2. _____

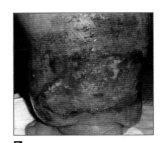

3. _____

A. Arterial ulcer

B. Lymphatic ulcer

C. Venous ulcer

My word!

Use the clues to help you unscramble the names of the major cause of each type of vascular ulcer. Then use the circled letters to answer the question posed.

Question: What is the most common type of vascular ulcer?

1. What disorder is the major cause of arterial ulcers?

cherriesalossto ___ ___ ___ ___ ___ ___ ___ ___ ___ ___ Ⓞ ___ ___ Ⓞ

2. What disorder is the major cause of venous ulcers?

conceiveiffunnyisus Ⓞ ___ ___ ___ Ⓞ ___ ___ Ⓞ ___ ___ ___ ___ ___ ___ ___

___ ___ ___ ___ ___

3. What disorder is the major cause of lymphatic ulcers?

playmedhem ___ ___ ___ ___ ___ Ⓞ ___ ___ ___ ___ ___

Selected References

Society for Vascular Surgery. (2014). Management of venous leg ulcers: Clinical practice guidelines of the Society for Vascular Surgery and the American Venous Forum. *Journal of Vascular Surgery, 60*(2, Suppl.), 3S–59S.

Wound, Ostomy, Continence Nurses Society. (2011). *Guideline for management of wounds in patients with lower-extremity arterial disease.* Mt. Laurel, NJ: Author.

Wound, Ostomy, Continence Nurses Society. (2011). *Guideline for management of wounds in patients with lower-extremity venous disease.* Mt. Laurel, NJ: Author.

Wound Healing Society. (2014). Wound Healing Society 2014 update on guidelines for arterial ulcers. *Wound Repair and Regeneration, 24,* 127–135.

Wound Healing Society. (2015). Wound Healing Society 2015 update on guidelines for arterial ulcers. *Wound Repair and Regeneration, 24,* 136–144.

Chapter 8

Diabetic foot ulcers

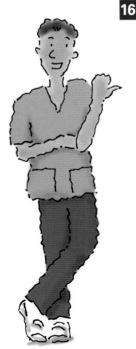

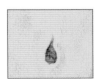

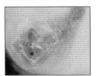

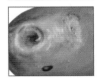

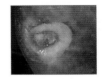

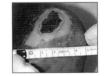

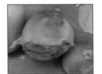

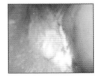

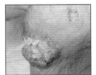

Causes

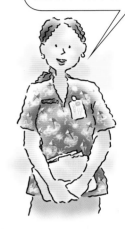

About 30 million adults and children in the United States have diabetes. Of those, between 19 and 34% will develop diabetic foot ulcers.

Diabetes mellitus—a metabolic disorder characterized by hyperglycemia—occurs because of a lack of insulin, a lack of insulin effect, or both. The high plasma glucose levels resulting from diabetes commonly damage blood vessels and nerves, leading to poor circulation and decreased sensation. This typically occurs in the lower extremities, leaving patients with diabetes at risk for developing foot ulcers.

Understanding diabetic neuropathy

Uncontrolled diabetes commonly results in three often concurrent types of neuropathy that dramatically increase a patient's risk of developing diabetic foot ulcers due to loss of protective sensation. Most diabetic foot ulcers are considered pressure injuries.

Neuropathy is a nerve disorder causing impaired or lost function in tissue served by affected nerve fibers. This disorder results in a loss of sensation, also referred to as **sensory neuropathy**, making the patient unaware of excessive pressure or friction (mechanical forces) that can lead to foot ulcers. Many patients with uncontrolled diabetes and neuropathy also have peripheral vascular disease and may not be aware that they have sensory neuropathy until they get a cut or blister on their foot or see blood in their shoe from trauma.

1 Sensory neuropathy

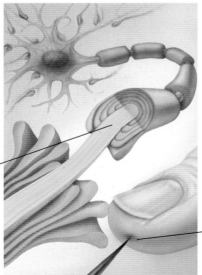

Ischemia or demyelination causes nerve death or deterioration...

...which results in decreased pain sensation.

2 Motor neuropathy

Motor neuropathy is also common in patients with diabetes. This disorder affects the nerves that innervate the muscles of the foot, resulting in weakness and often a change in the shape of the foot and toes (i.e., claw foot or hammer toes.)

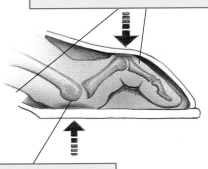

Muscular atrophy in the plantar surface of the foot results in increased arch height and clawed toes.

In addition, the fat pad that normally covers the metatarsal heads thins and migrates toward the toes, exposing the heads to pressure and increasing ulcer risk.

3 Autonomic neuropathy

Autonomic neuropathy results when nerves are damaged that affect bodily functions. In the feet, skin becomes dry, flaky, and cracked, especially around the heels, due to loss of function of the sweat and oil glands, and the toenails can become thick and discolored.

In Charcot's disease, bones weakened by osteopenia suffer fractures that the patient doesn't feel because of sensory neuropathy. Over time, this process causes bony destruction that culminates with the collapse of the midfoot into a rocker bottom deformity.

In uncontrolled diabetes, autonomic neuropathy inhibits or destroys the sympathetic component of the autonomic nervous system, which controls vasoconstriction in peripheral blood vessels. The resulting unrestricted flow of blood to the lower limbs and feet may cause osteopenia in foot and ankle bones.

Midfoot ulcers that result from increased plantar pressure over the rocker bottom deformity heal more slowly than ulcers on the forefoot.

Performing the Semmes-Weinstein test for neuropathy

In the Semmes-Weinstein test, the practitioner uses a special monofilament to assess protective sensation in the feet of a patient with diabetes. This test helps to identify the degree of sensory neuropathy.

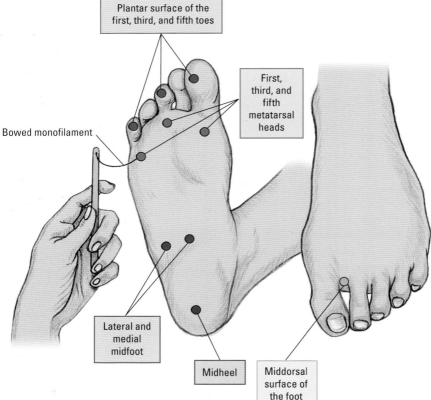

Plantar surface of the first, third, and fifth toes

First, third, and fifth metatarsal heads

Bowed monofilament

Lateral and medial midfoot

Midheel

Middorsal surface of the foot

Performing the test
- Ask the patient to close his eyes.
- Ask the patient to identify where and when he feels the monofilament touch.
- Place the 10-g monofilament on one of the testing points shown at right, and exert enough pressure to bow the monofilament. Count to one and release.

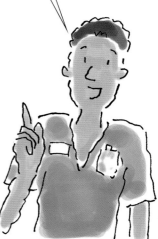

When performing the Semmes-Weinstein test, the monofilament should bow as shown in this illustration.

Characteristics

Diabetic foot ulcers, also called neuropathic ulcers, commonly develop under a bony prominence, such as the one shown here under the metatarsal head of the great toe. Other common sites are under the first, third, and fifth metatarsal heads just below the crease of the toes. Often a thick callus precedes the ulcer, but not always. Ulcers can have callused skin around them.

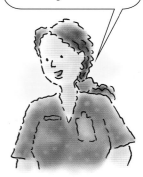

Impaired circulation and sensory neuropathy set the stage for ulcers to develop. These conditions allow excessive, repetitive pressure on the soles of the feet to go unchecked, commonly leading to an ulcer.

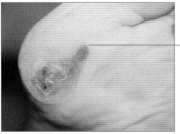

Small blood streaks indicate tissue trauma. This callus should be watched carefully as it could open into an ulcer.

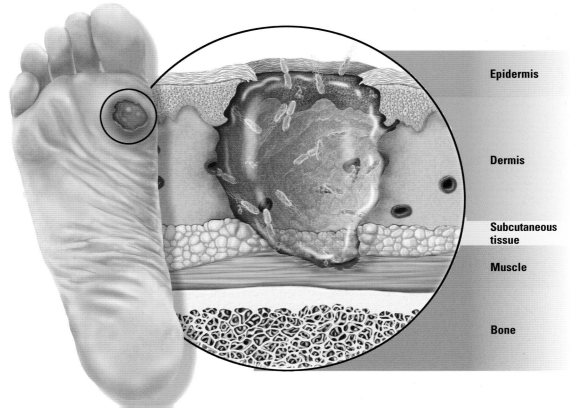

Epidermis

Dermis

Subcutaneous tissue

Muscle

Bone

Characteristics of skin surrounding a diabetic foot ulcer

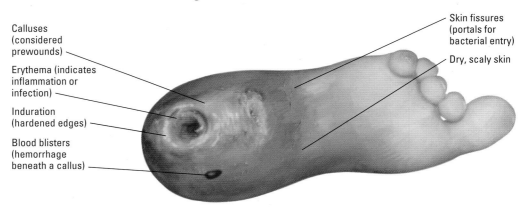

Calluses (considered prewounds)

Erythema (indicates inflammation or infection)

Induration (hardened edges)

Blood blisters (hemorrhage beneath a callus)

Skin fissures (portals for bacterial entry)

Dry, scaly skin

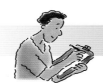

Take note

Documenting a diabetic foot ulcer

2/28/18 1430 Dressing changed on diabetic foot ulcer on Ⓛ heel. Ulcer measures 2 cm length, 3 cm width, and 0.5 cm depth. No drainage or odor noted. Pedal pulses palpable. Patient unable to feel monofilament under great toe, and all metatarsal heads. Site cleaned with NSS and allowed to dry thoroughly. Wound bed appears moist and pink with a thin ring of yellow slough at edges. Calloused border noted at wound edge from 6 o'clock to 8 o'clock. Hydrogel applied to site and dressed per physician order. Maintaining heels off bed, using heel elevator device. Ambulated with special orthotic shoe to off-load pressure. Tolerated procedure well; rates pain as 1 on a 0-to-10 scale before and after procedure. ——— *Diane Bettick, R.N.*

Ulcer location	Characteristics
Plantar surface	Even wound margins
Great toe	Deep wound bed
Metatarsal head	Dry or low to moderate exudate
Heel	Low to moderate exudate
Tip or top of toe	Pale granulation tissue with ischemia or bright red, friable granulation tissue with infection

A closer look at diabetic foot ulcers

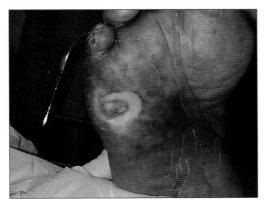

This photo shows a diabetic foot ulcer on the plantar surface of the fifth metatarsal head. The circular shape of the wound is consistent with a wound created by pressure over a bony prominence.

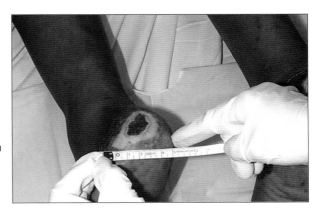

This photo shows a pressure injury that has developed over the heel from impaired protective sensation and poor mobility.

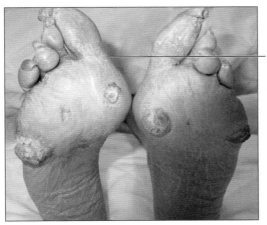

Sensory neuropathy can lead to excessive callus formation. This patient was unaware of the callus.

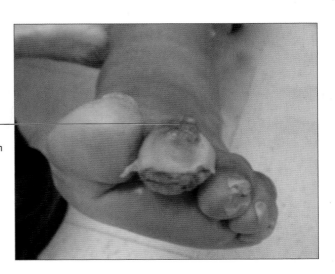

Ulcers can hide under whitish tissue such as this one. The circulation in this toe was poor, leading to eventual toe amputation.

Classification

> Classifying diabetic ulcers helps ensure that all members of the health care team provide treatment appropriate to the ulcer's severity.

Depending on the classification system, diabetic foot ulcers are classified according to depth, presence of ischemia, and presence of infection.

University of Texas Diabetic Foot Classification System

The University of Texas Diabetic Foot Classification System provides a detailed categorization, which includes infection and ischemia.

Stage	Grade 0	Grade I	Grade II	Grade III
A	Preulcerative or postulcerative foot at risk for further ulceration	Superficial ulcer without tendon, capsule, or bone involvement	Ulcer penetrating to tendon or joint capsule	Ulcer penetrating to bone
B	Presence of infection	Presence of infection	Presence of infection	Presence of infection
C	Presence of ischemia	Presence of ischemia	Presence of ischemia	Presence of ischemia
D	Presence of infection and ischemia	Presence of infection and ischemia	Presence of infection and ischemia	Presence of infection and ischemia

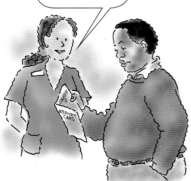

> This isn't like in school. In this instance, a low score is a good thing.

Wagner Ulcer Grade Classification

In the Wagner Ulcer Grade Classification, less complex ulcers receive lower scores; more complex ulcers, higher scores. Ulcers with higher scores may require surgical intervention or amputation.

Grade	Characteristics
0	• Preulcerous lesion • Healed ulcer • Presence of bony deformity
1	• Superficial ulcer without subcutaneous tissue involvement
2	• Penetration through the subcutaneous tissue; may expose bone, tendon, ligament, or joint capsule
3	• Osteitis, abscess, or osteomyelitis
4	• Gangrene of a digit
5	• Gangrene requiring foot amputation

Treatment

Successful ulcer healing depends on proper wound care and off-loading. The care plan may also include debridement, antimicrobials, biotherapies, and surgery.

Treatment algorithm for diabetic ulcers

- Establish etiology.
- Review past medical treatments.
- Review medication history.
- Perform noninvasive vascular assessment.
- Evaluate the patient's footwear.

Ischemic: Ankle-brachial index < 0.8
Vascular consult (if indicated)

Neuropathic: Ankle-brachial index > 0.9
Assess degree of neuropathy

Debridement

Ischemic, stable
- Nonaggressive dressing treatment

Nonischemic, neuropathic
- Debride hyperkeratotic rim
- Perform aggressive sharp debridement

Infection?

Yes   No   Yes

Localized soft tissue
- Broad-spectrum oral antibiotics
- Reevaluation in 1 week
- Non-weight-bearing activity (if possible)
- Control of diabetes

Wound care

Localized bone; systemic
- Admission to hospital
- Appropriate cultures
- I.V. antibiotics
- Possibly, surgical intervention

Wound care algorithm for diabetic ulcers

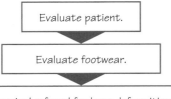

| Evaluate patient. |

| Evaluate footwear. |

| Surgical referral for bony deformities |

Wagner Grade 0	**Wagner Grade 1**	**Wagner Grade 2**	**Wagner Grade 3**	**Wagner Grades 4 and 5**
■ Padding and accommodative devices ■ Callus debridement	■ Follow grade 0 protocol ■ Topical antiseptics on highly contaminated wounds ■ Nonocclusive dressing ■ Weekly evaluation until healed ■ Plantar surface—foam dressing ■ Dorsal surface—occlusive or nonocclusive dressing	■ Follow grade 1 protocol ■ Rule out osteomyelitis (X-ray, bone scan, bone biopsy, or MRI) ■ Non–weight-bearing activity ■ Surgical consult ■ Plantar surface—amorphous hydrogel/hydrofiber, alginate, or foam dressing ■ Dorsal surface—occlusive dressing if no drainage ■ Topical antimicrobial cream, ointment, or amorphous hydrogel	■ Follow grade 1 protocol ■ Rule out osteomyelitis (X-ray, bone scan, bone biopsy, or MRI) ■ Plantar surface—amorphous hydrogel/hydrofiber, alginate, or foam dressing ■ Dorsal surface—nonocclusive dressing ■ Topical antimicrobial cream, ointment, or amorphous hydrogel Advanced wound healing technologies might be prescribed	■ Surgical consult and intervention

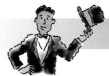

Best dressed

Dressings for diabetic foot ulcers

Type of ulcer	Recommended dressings
Dry	• Hydrogel/hydrofiber
Wet	• Alginate • Foam • Collagen
Shallow	• Transparent film • Hydrocolloid
Tunneling or deep	• Alginate ropes (for wet ulcers) • Hydrogel impregnated strip gauze(for dry ulcers)
Infected	• Iodosorb or Iodoflex (cadexomer iodine products absorbing fluid, exudate, and bacteria) • Products with an antimicrobial component
Bleeding	• Alginate

Off-loading

Patients with diabetic neuropathy no longer feel the pressure or pain that normally precedes tissue damage. Therefore, relieving pressure from plantar tissues—known as *off-loading*—is key to treating and preventing ulcers. Off-loading can be accomplished using nonsurgical and surgical interventions.

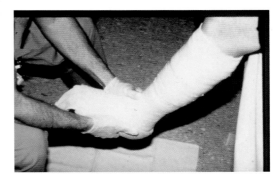

Nonsurgical interventions
• Therapeutic footwear (possibly with rocker soles)

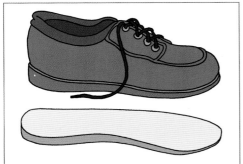

This shoe has a toe box with extra depth and width to accommodate bony deformities, such as claw toes and hallux valgus (displacement of the great toe toward other toes). The shoe can also be modified to allow room for a widened hindfoot/heel. The soft, thick inlay provides comfort and protection.

Surgical interventions
• Exostectomy
• Digital arthroplasty
• Bone and joint resections
• Partial calcanectomy

• Custom orthotics
• Walking casts (such as a total contact cast)
• Walkers
• Splints

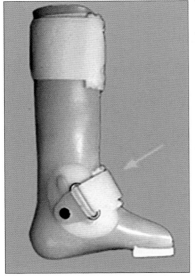

This ankle-foot orthosis is used to relieve pressure from the heel.

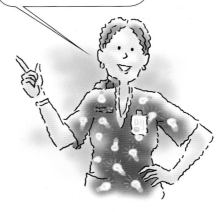

Keep in mind that using an off-loading device can increase the patient's risk of falling. Be sure to teach the patient about fall prevention. Physical therapy is helpful for gait training.

Prevention

Diabetic ulcer prevention starts with teaching patients how to control diabetes and how to care for their feet.

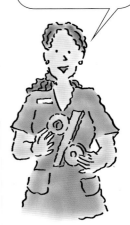

Comprehensive foot care programs can reduce ulcer-related amputation rates by up to 50%.

Maceration leads to skin breakdown as well as fungal infections.

Teaching topic	Teaching tips
Diabetes control	• Emphasize the importance of controlling diabetes. Discuss the consequences of failing to control diabetes (such as peripheral neuropathy and vascular damage). • Explain that careful glycemic control (by monitoring Hb A_{1c} levels at regular intervals) can reduce the frequency and severity of neuropathy in people with type 1 or type 2 diabetes.
Foot hygiene	• Check feet daily for injury or pressure areas (using a long-handled mirror may make viewing easier). • Wash feet with a mild soap, and dry thoroughly between the toes. • Before getting in, check bath water to make sure it isn't too hot. (Test the water with an elbow, use a thermometer, or ask a family member to help.) • Apply a moisturizing cream to feet to prevent dry, cracked skin and to balance skin pH. Don't apply moisturizer between the toes. • Cut toenails off squarely and smooth the ragged corners with a nail file. Consult a podiatrist if toenails are deformed and thickened. • Don't go barefooted; the risk of injury is too great.
Choosing socks	• Wear white or light-colored socks to make bleeding from trauma easy to detect. • Wear socks that fit well, not too loose or tight, and not too short in the toes. • Choose socks that wick perspiration away from the feet to prevent maceration. • Use diabetic padded socks for shear and friction control but make sure that shoes are big enough to accommodate the thicker socks.
Choosing shoes	• Wear shoes that fit well, not shoes that are too tight or loose. • Wear shoes that breathe to reduce maceration and fungal infections. • Wear new shoes for short periods (<1 hour) each day initially; gradually increase the time as your feet adjust. • If you have any foot deformities or have a history of ulceration, wear professionally fitted shoes. • If possible, wash your shoes to destroy microorganisms. • Check your shoes before putting them on to make sure that they don't contain anything that could cause an injury.

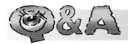

Show and tell

Describe the pathophysiology of sensory neuropathy illustrated here.

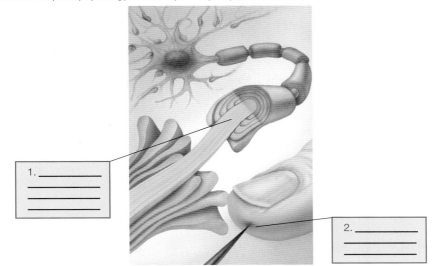

1. _____

2. _____

1. _____
_____
_____

2. _____
_____

Able to label?

Identify the bony abnormalities associated with diabetic motor neuropathy on this illustration.

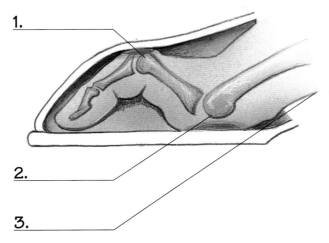

1. _____

2. _____

3. _____

Answers: Show and tell 1. Ischemia or demyelination causes nerve death or deterioration, 2. Decreased pain sensation results; Able to label? 1. Clawed toes, 2. Downward displacement of the metatarsal heads, 3. Increased arch height.

Selected References

American Diabetes Association. (2016). Microvascular complications and foot care. *Diabetes Care, 39*(Suppl. 1), S72–S80. https://doi.org/10.2337/dc16-S012

Infectious Diseases Society of America. (2012). 2012 Infectious Diseases Society of America Clinical Practice Guideline for the diagnosis and treatment of diabetic foot infections. Infectious Diseases Society of America. http://cid.oxfordjournals.org

Wounds International. (2013). Best practice guidelines: Wound management in diabetic foot ulcers. www.woundsinternational.com

Wound, Ostomy, Continence Nurses Society. (2012). Guideline for management of wounds in patients with lower-extremity neuropathic disease. Mt. Laurel, NJ: Author.

Chapter 9

Malignant wounds

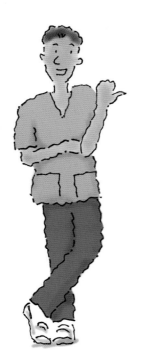

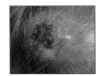

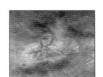

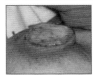

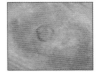

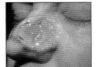

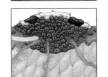

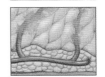

Causes

Malignant wounds may be due to cancer of the skin or develop when a primary or metastatic tumor infiltrates the epidermis. Occurring in 5% to 10% of cancer patients, these wounds grow rapidly and commonly invade surrounding tissues and organs, sometimes creating sinus tracts and fistulas. Malignant wounds can have an ulcerated or a cauliflower-like appearance; they are poorly perfused with friable, fragile blood vessels and contain large amounts of necrotic tissue. The most common locations for malignant wounds are the head, neck, and chest.

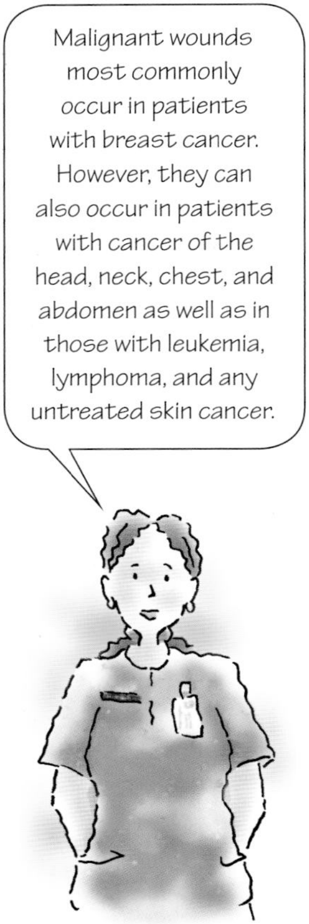

Malignant wounds most commonly occur in patients with breast cancer. However, they can also occur in patients with cancer of the head, neck, chest, and abdomen as well as in those with leukemia, lymphoma, and any untreated skin cancer.

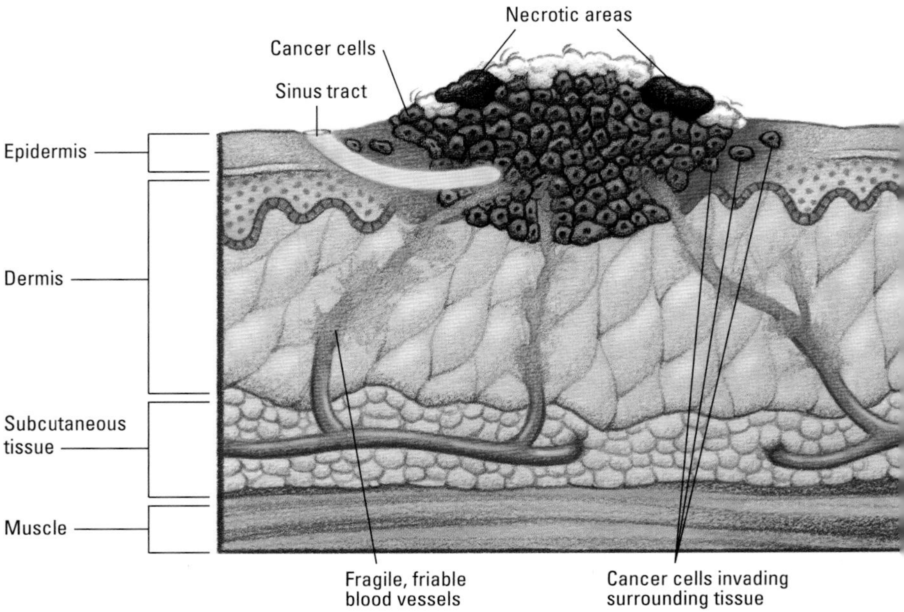

Necrotic areas

Cancer cells

Sinus tract

Epidermis

Dermis

Subcutaneous tissue

Muscle

Fragile, friable blood vessels

Cancer cells invading surrounding tissue

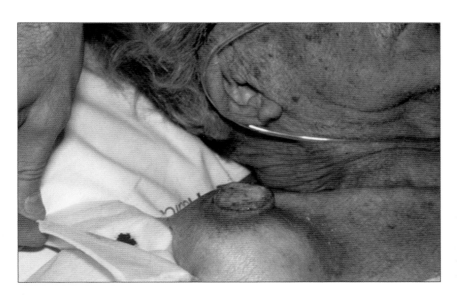

◄ This squamous cell carcinoma, after being neglected, ulcerated to form the malignant wound shown here.

This basal cell carcinoma was also neglected. It eventually ulcerated and invaded deeper tissue. ►

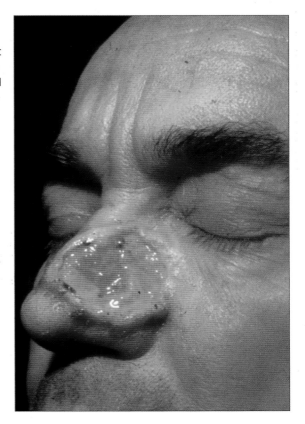

Malignant wounds can develop from a skin cancer that has not been treated or has recurred.

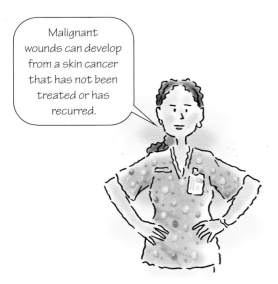

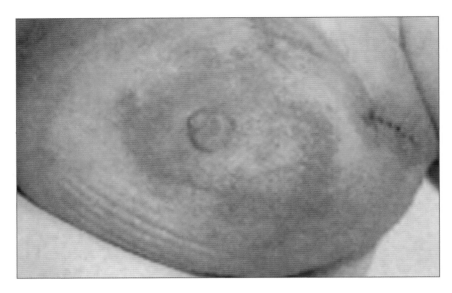

◀ This photo shows an inflamed carcinoma of the breast.

The malignant wound shown here resulted when a lymphoma metastasized to the patient's scalp ▶

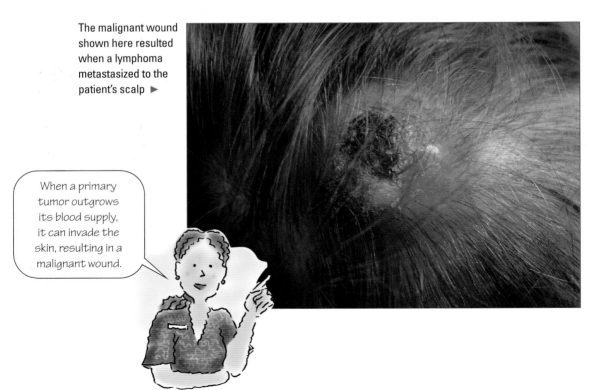

When a primary tumor outgrows its blood supply, it can invade the skin, resulting in a malignant wound.

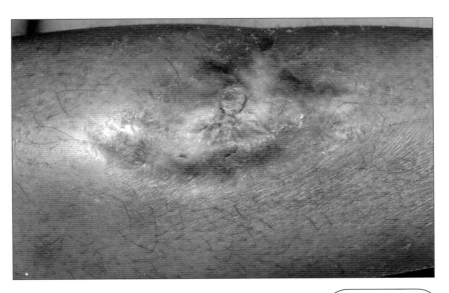

◄ This photo shows a squamous cell carcinoma arising from a burn scar.

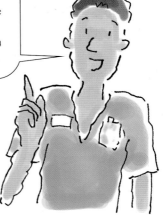

Chronic wounds, or even scar tissue, can evolve into a malignant wound. This type of malignant wound is called a Marjolin's ulcer.

Complications

Problem	Causes	Management strategies
Odor	Nonviable, necrotic tissue and excessive drainage create an ideal environment for bacterial growth. In turn, this produces a foul odor. Polymicrobial bacteria are responsible for causing odor. Odor-causing bacteria can be aerobic such as, *Klebsiella*, *Proteus*, *Pseudomonas*, and *Staphylococcus*, or they can be anaerobic such as *Clostridium* and *Bacteroides fragilis*. Odor can cause nausea, vomiting, and loss of appetite for the patient.	• Change dressings and gently irrigate the wound with tap water or normal saline solution at frequent intervals. • Apply topical antibiotics to reduce the amount of bacteria. • Foam, calcium alginate, hydrofiber, composite, and occlusive dressings may be used based on wound characteristics. See chapter 11 for more on dressings. • Use other topical antimicrobials, such as metronidazole gel or crushed metronidazole tablets, Iodoflex or Iodosorb, or silver-containing products, as indicated. • Antiseptic solutions such as acetic acid or sodium hypochlorite can reduce odor but might sting and require at least daily dressing changes. • Use charcoal dressings, such as Carbonet, CarboFlex, and Actisorb Plus. • Room deodorizers and odor masking techniques can be helpful such as: • Peppermint, lavender, or lemon scents. • Apply Mentholatum (Vicks VapoRub) near the patient's or caregiver's nostrils to minimize the perception of odor. • Place a tray of kitty litter, baking soda, or charcoal under the patient's bed to absorb odors. • Room ventilation. • Apply a pouching system to the wound to help control odors.
Bleeding	Malignant cells stimulate angiogenesis. Thrombocytopenia and disseminated intravascular coagulopathy and malnutrition are factors common in cancer patients, leading to increased vascular permeability and promote a loss of protein and fibrinogen. This causes the blood vessels surrounding a malignant wound to become friable and fragile, and the blood to have an impaired ability to clot.	• Use nonadherent or low adhesive dressings (such as silicone dressings) to minimize tissue trauma and reduce the risk of bleeding. • Avoid frequent or unnecessary dressing changes. • For small bleeding areas, consider using alginate dressings and/or hemostatic agents (such as Gelfoam, Surgicel, Spongostan, silver nitrate, and Oxycel) • For larger areas, epinephrine soaked gauze can be applied in layers • Assist with surgical intervention (cauterization) or the application of topical epinephrine (Adrenalin) 1:1,000 to control profuse bleeding. • Administer oral antifibrinolytics (such as tranexamic acid [Cyklokapron] or aminocaproic acid [Amicar]), as prescribed, to control severe bleeding.

Problem	Causes	Management strategies
Exudate (drainage)	The leakage of fibrinogen and plasma colloids by vessels in the wound causes exudate to form. Bacteria in the wound release enzymes that liquefy tissue, producing additional exudate.	• Use highly absorbent dressings (such as calcium alginate, foam, and hydrofiber) in wounds with moderate to large amounts of exudate. • Administer topical or systemic antimicrobials, as prescribed, to reduce bacterial load and exudate. • Use a wound drainage system, such as a pouch, on wounds with large amounts of exudate. (Avoid using a negative pressure system.) • Protect the surrounding skin from maceration and irritation. • Use stockinette, tube sleeves, and binders when possible to secure dressings and minimize tape to skin.
Pruritus (itching)	Edema, bacteria, and tumor all cause cellular inflammation and destruction. This causes the skin to stretch and the peripheral nerves become irritated, commonly resulting in pruritus. Fungal infections may also cause pruritus.	• Chill emollients, hydrogel sheet dressings, and other topically applied agents in the refrigerator and then apply to the wound. • Apply menthol creams to the affected area. • Advise the patient to use cool or lukewarm water to bath or shower, rather than hot water. • Advise the patient that antihistamines may only have a limited effect on the pruritus associated with malignant wounds. • Administer oral medications such as gabapentin, doxepin, or mirtazapine as ordered. • Topical agents such as tacrolimus, lidocaine applied before capsaician (to reduce stinging), and topical cannabinoid agonist agents can offer temporary relief.
Pain	Pressure on nerve endings from edema and the tumor as well as exposure of the dermis to air may cause chronic pain. Dressing changes and other procedures may also worsen pain.	• Use a reliable and valid pain assessment tool—such as the visual analog, numeric pain intensity, or FACES pain-rating scales—to accurately assess the patient's level of pain. • Determine triggering and relieving factors. • Administer prescribed pain medication (oral or parenteral) or topical anesthetics as ordered and before changing dressings or performing procedures. • Allow for 'time-out' if dressing change is too painful. • Nonadhesive dressings may be more comfortable.

Treatment

The goal behind any wound management system is to protect the wound and the surrounding areas and to provide an ideal environment for healing. However, because malignant wounds tend to occur near the end of a patient's life, treatment typically focuses on minimizing complications, controlling symptoms, and offering psychological support rather than on healing.

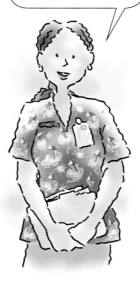

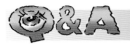

Matchmaker

Match the five complications of malignant wounds shown on the left with the management strategies shown on the right.

1. Odor _____

2. Bleeding _____

3. Exudate _____

4. Pruritus _____

5. Pain _____

A. Administer analgesics as ordered.

B. Use nonadherent dressings.

C. Apply topical antimicrobials to the wound.

D. Use a wound drainage system such as a pouch.

E. Apply cooled hydrogel sheets to the wound.

Best answer

What is the primary goal of topical care for malignant wound?

1. Diagnosing the wound

2. Minimize complications

3. Heal the wound

4. Manage odor

Which of the following is best to manage a heavily draining malignant breast wound?

1. Chilled hydrogel sheet

2. Silver nitrate application

3. Alginate and foam dressing

4. Metronidazole gel and gauze dressing

Selected References

Alexander, S. (2009). Malignant fungating wounds: Epidemiology, aetiology, presentation and assessment. *Journal of Wound Care, 18*(7), 273–280.

Bergstrom, K. J. (2011). Assessment and management of fungating wounds. *Journal of Wound, Ostomy, and Continence Nursing, 38*(1), 31–37.

Emmons, K., & Dale, B. (2016). Palliative wound care. In D. Doughty, & L. McNichol, (Eds.), *Wound, Ostomy and Continence Nurses Society (2016). Core Curriculum: Wound Management* (pp. 690–703). Philadelphia, PA: Wolters Kluwer.

Fromantin, I., Watson, S., Baffie, A., Rivat, A., Falcou, M., Kriegel, I., & de Rycke Ingenior, Y. (2014). A prospective, descriptive cohort study of malignant wound characteristics and wound care strategies in patients with breast cancer. *Ostomy Wound Management, 60*(6), 38–48.

Ghasemi, F., Anooshirvani, N., Sibbald, R. G., & Alavi, A. (2016). The point prevalence of malignancy in a wound clinic. *International Journal of Lower Extremity Wounds, 15*(1), 58–62. doi:10.1177/1534734615627721

Ladizinski, B., Alavi, A., Jambrosic, J., Mistry, N., & Sibbald, R. G. (2014). Cancers mimicking fungal infections. *Advances in Skin and Wound Care, 27*(7), 301–305. doi:10.1097/01.ASW.0000446864.26807.43

O'Brien, C. (2012). Malignant wounds: Managing odour. *Canadian Family Physician, 58*(3), 272–274.

Recka, K., Montagnini, M., & Vitale, C. A. (2012). Management of bleeding associated with malignant wounds. *Journal of Palliative Medicine, 15*(8), 952–954. doi:10.1089/jpm.2011.0286

Scheer, H. S., Kaiser, M., & Zingg, U. (2017). Results of directly applied activated carbon cloth in chronic wounds: A preliminary study. *Journal of Wound Care, 26*(8), 476–481. doi:10.12968/jowc.2017.26.8.476

Vasques, C. I., & Sacramento, C. (2015). Management of signs and symptoms in malignant wounds: An integrative review. *Cancer Nursing, 38*, S87–S88.

Young, T. (2017). Caring for patients with malignant and end-of-life wounds. *Wounds UK, 13*, 20–29.

Atypical wounds

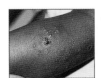

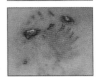

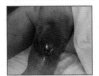

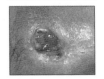

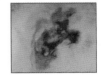

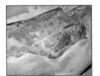

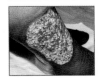

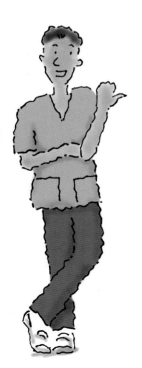

Causes

External causes
- Bites
- Radiation
- Trauma
- Chemical

Metabolic and autoimmune disorders
- Calciphylaxis
- Epidermolysis bullosa
- Sickle cell anemia
- Antiphospholipid antibody syndrome
- Systemic lupus erythematosus
- Scleroderma

Inflammatory processes
- Pyoderma gangrenosum
- Vasculitis
- Intertrigo

Neoplasms
- Basal cell carcinoma
- Kaposi's sarcoma
- Lymphoma
- Squamous cell carcinoma
- Melanoma

Infection
- Atypical mycobacteria
- Fungal infections
- Necrotizing fasciitis

Types

External causes

Bites, such as those from insects and animals, are one type of atypical wound.

Erythematous lesion with central eschar caused by a spider bite

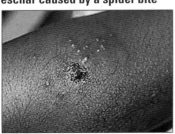

Wounds from several dog bites

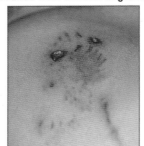

Blunt trauma is common in the elderly

Bullae from trauma.

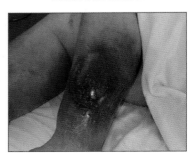

Intertrigo

Intertrigo is the inflammation of a skinfold or two areas of skin that rub together.

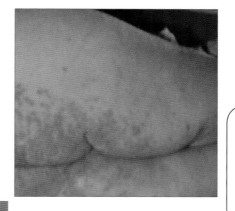

> Intertrigo can occur in any skinfold but is most prevalent under the breasts, in the pannus (abdominal skinfolds), and in the axillary, submaxillary, groin, and perineal areas.

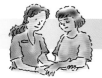

Special attention

Intertrigo in bariatric patients

Bariatric patients are at higher risk for developing intertriginous dermatitis (dermatitis that occurs between skinfolds) because multiple large skinfolds create conditions that are perfect for infection and inflammation. These conditions include:

* pressure of large skinfolds on underlying skin, creating pressure-induced injury
* moisture (perspiration is trapped under skinfolds, resulting in maceration)
* friction
* shear with movement, resulting in fissures
* physical challenges in maintaining hygiene
* warm, dark, and moist conditions that favor the growth of yeast and fungi.

Intravenous extravasation ulcers

Chronic ulceration from chemotherapy infiltration

Extravasation is the unintentional administration of a vesicant, irritant, or nonvesicant solution into surrounding tissue. This is an example of chemical wounds. Vesicants (chemotherapy agents, certain electrolyte solutions, radiographic contrast media, and vasopressors) are solutions capable of causing tissue injury or destruction for an extended period of time. Irritants and nonvesicants such as alkylating agents, carmustine, or vincristine can also be destructive but these tend to be excreted more quickly.

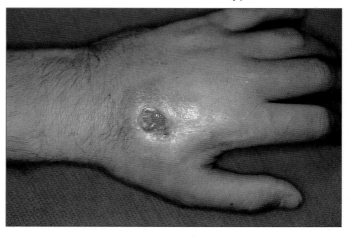

Necrotizing fasciitis

Necrotizing fasciitis is a severe potentially life-threatening type of infection in which bacteria enter the body through a minor wound and release harmful toxins that interfere with the tissue's blood supply. Extensive tissue damage often occurs under the skin. It starts with tenderness.

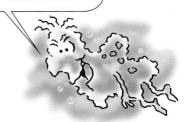

Once my friends and I spread, necrotizing fasciitis can quickly lead to death.

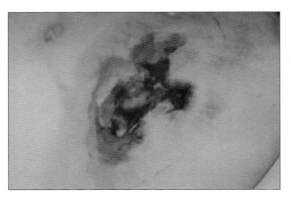

Classic signs
1. Warm skin, and a painful bump or spot on the skin
2. Typically, a bronze or purple-colored blister forms with a rapidly spreading area of erythema. Tissue necrosis progresses with gangrene of the area

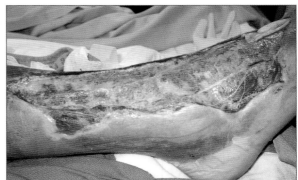

Pyoderma gangrenosum ulcers

Pyoderma gangrenosum ulcers are examples of wound due to imflammatory processes. The ulcerative type occurs most commonly on the legs after injury or trauma. The atypical type of pyoderma gangrenosum occurs on the torso and upper limbs. Often multiple small pustular or bullous lesions merge into one large ulcer.

Painful, open ulcer with reddish-purple irregular borders

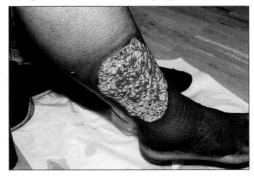

Scleroderma

The word scleroderma means thickening of the skin. In this autoimmune disease, fibrosis occurs most commonly on the hands but can also be seen on the face, neck, and upper chest.

Acrocyanosis and ulcer formation in scleroderma

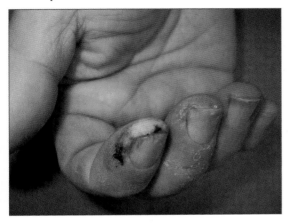

Systemic lupus erythematosus ulcers

Systemic lupus erythematosus (SLE) ulcers most commonly occur on the scalp and face and sometimes look like psoriasis.

SLE ulcers can be aggravated by sunlight and other ultraviolet light.

Red, scaly SLE ulcer

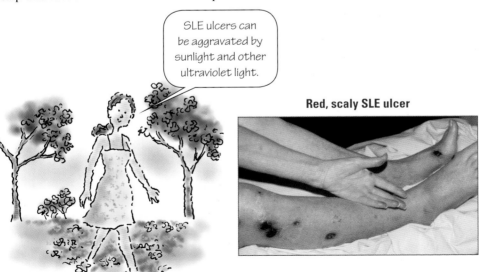

Thromboangiitis obliterans

Also known as *Buerger's disease*, is a rare form of vasculitis that affects the arteries and the veins. It is an inflammatory condition that leads to thrombosis in some superficial veins and small- and medium-sized arteries. It causes arterial ischemia in distal extremities and superficial thrombophlebitis.

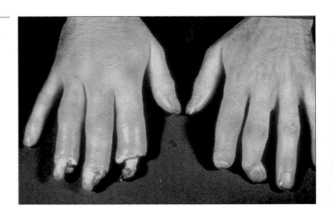

Necrotic drug eruptions—these can include heparin- and warfarin-induced necrosis

For injectable anticoagulants, the necrosis occurs at the site of infusion or injection, for warfarin (Coumadin)-induced necrosis commonly occurs on the breasts, buttocks, thighs, and abdomen.

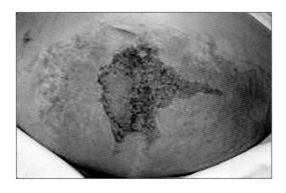

The abundance of small dermal blood vessels in fatty tissue may explain why warfarin-induced necrosis is more common in some areas.

Neoplasms

Nonmelanoma skin cancers, basal cell and squamous cell carcinomas, are the most common types of skin cancers. Kaposi's sarcoma, lymphomas, and melanoma are less common but all can present as atypical wounds. Establishing the diagnosis requires a skin biopsy and is essential to determining the treatment.

This is a squamous cell carcinoma, note the red base and horn-like appearance in the center

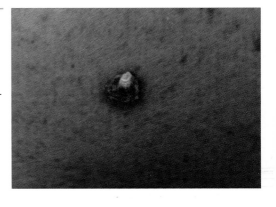

Treatments

Black widow spider bite
* Immediate medical attention
* Cool compresses
* Elevation, if possible
* Antivenom
* Calcium gluconate
* Antihistamines
* Analgesics
* Local wound care with nonadhesive or low adhesive dressings to minimize pain

Brown recluse spider bite
* Cool compresses
* Elevation, if possible
* Analgesics
* Systemic corticosteroids
* Aggressive local wound care
* Debridement
* Grafting

Dog bite
* Antibiotics
* Rabies therapy
* Tetanus vaccination
* Local wound care with nonadhesive or low adhesive dressings to minimize pain
* Topical steroids may be needed to manage intense itch
* Debridement and grafting, if the wound is extensive

Intertrigo
* Eliminating friction, heat, and maceration by keeping skinfolds cool and dry
* Moisture wicking textiles such as InterDry Ag
* Antimycotic agents (nystatin)
* Protective barrier ointments

I.V. extravasation ulcers
* Immediate cessation of the infusion
* Flushing of the area with normal saline solution within 24 hours
* Local infiltration of the affected area with dilute antidote (varies depending on the drug extravasated)
* Debridement and topical care, depending on wound characteristics
* Grafting
* Possible amputation, if gangrene results

Necrotizing fasciitis
* Frequent surgical debridement
* Broad-spectrum antibiotics
* Grafting or flap
* Aggressive local wound care

* Negative pressure wound therapy
* Local wound care—if extensive dressing changes may need to be done under anesthesia

Pyoderma gangrenosum ulcers
* Systemic management of underlying disease
* Corticosteroids (topical, systemic, intralesional)
* Immunosuppressive agents such as cyclosporine (systemic, topical)
* Antimicrobial agents, such as tetracycline and vancomycin
* Antitumor necrosis factor (alpha) medications, such as infliximab (Remicade) and etanercept (Enbrel)
* Blood products
* Immunomodulators, such as I.V. immunoglobulin (IVIG)
* Hyperbaric oxygen
* Local wound care with low adhesive dressings such as with foams, gels, and silicone dressings

Scleroderma
* Systemic management of underlying disease
* Nitrates, such as nitroglycerin, for vasodilation
* Debridement
* Hyperbaric oxygen therapy
* Local wound care—nonocclusive dressings with nonadhesive or low adhesive surfaces, commonly treated like vascular wounds

SLE ulcers
* Systemic management of underlying disease
* Corticosteroids (systemic, topical)
* Immunosuppressants (such as azathioprine [Imuran] or cyclophosphamide [Cytoxan])
* Hyperbaric oxygen therapy
* Local wound care

Thromboangiitis obliterans
* Smoking abstinence (cornerstone of treatment)
* Calcium channel blockers such as nifedipine (Procardia)
* Arterial bypass
* Major or minor amputations
* Avoidance of cold temperatures
* Aspirin
* Vasodilators
* Surgical sympathectomy for pain management

Warfarin (Coumadin)-induced necrosis
* Discontinuation of warfarin
* I.V. heparin
* Debridement
* Grafting
* Muscle flaps

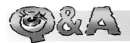

Matchmaker

Match the atypical wounds shown at right with their names.

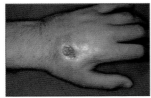

1. _____

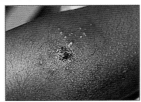

2. _____

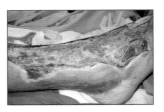

3. _____

A. Necrotizing fasciitis

B. Spider bite

C. Intravenous extravasation ulcer

My word!

Use the clues to help you unscramble three terms related to atypical wounds. Then use the circled letters to answer the question posed.

Question: Intertrigo is the term used to describe inflammation of a what?

1. A brand name for warfarin

   aimnocud   __ ◯ __ __ __ ◯ __ __

2. Type of anemia that is one cause of atypical wounds

   kslice lecl   ◯ __ __ ◯ __ __ __ __ __ ◯

3. Type of infection in which bacteria release toxins that interfere with the tissue's blood supply

   zircontinge isifcatis   ◯ __ __ __ __ __ __ __ ◯ __ __ ◯ __

Answer: ___ __ __ __ __ __ __

Best answer

Determining the cause of an atypical wound is critical because:

1. Wound care and dressing costs can vary
2. Accurate documentation is needed for billing
3. Some wounds cannot heal
4. Wound care for one wound may be contraindicated in another wound

Which of the following conditions most commonly occur on the hands?

1. Thromboangiitis obliterans
2. Pyoderma gangrenosa
3. Warfarin induced necrosis
4. Necrotizing fasciitis

Best answer: 4. 1.

Answers: Matchmaker 1. C, 2. B, 3. A; My word! 1. Coumadin, 2. Sickle cell, 3. Necrotizing fasciitis;

Selected References

Agarwal, A., Cardones, A. R., & Bauer, C. (2016). Wounds caused by dermatologic conditions. In D. Doughty & L. McNichol (Eds.), *Wound, Ostomy and Continence Nurses Society (2016). Core curriculum: Wound management* (pp. 573–586). Philadelphia, PA: Wolters Kluwer.

Bauer, C. (2016). Oncology-related skin and wound care. In D. Doughty & L. McNichol (Eds.), *Wound, Ostomy and Continence Nurses Society (2016). Core curriculum: Wound management* (pp. 587–610). Philadelphia, PA: Wolters Kluwer.

Blackett, A, Camden, S. G., Dungan, S., et al. (2011). Caring for persons with bariatric health care issues: A primer for the WOC Nurse. *Journal of Wound, Ostomy, and Continence Nursing, 38*(2), 133–140.

Distler, O., & Cozzio, A. (2016). Systemic sclerosis and localized scleroderma—current concepts and novel targets for therapy. *Seminars in Immunopathology, 38*(1), 87–95. doi:10.1007/s00281-015-0551-z

Kucisec-Tepes, N. (2013). Atypical wounds. *EWMA Journal, 13*(1), 86–87.

Ratnagobal, S., & Sinha, S. (2013). Pyoderma gangrenosum: Guideline for wound practitioners. *Journal of Wound Care, 22*(2), 68–73.

Van Driessche, F. (2016). Wounds caused by infectious processe. In D. Doughty & L. McNichol (Eds.), *Wound, Ostomy and Continence Nurses Society (2016). Core curriculum: Wound management* (pp. 558–574). Philadelphia, PA: Wolters Kluwer.

Watkins, J. (2016). Diagnosis, treatment and management of epidermolysis bullosa. *British Journal of Nursing, 25*(8), 428–431.

Chapter 11

Wound care products

 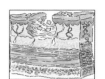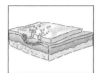
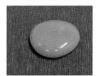

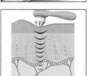

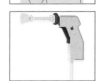

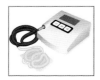

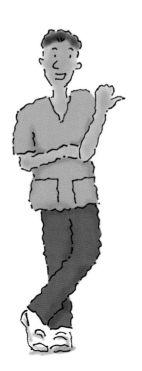

Development of wound care products

Over time, wound care has evolved from a fairly rudimentary practice that focused primarily on the injury to a process that takes the patient's overall health into account.

Dressings

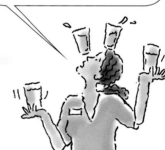

Controlling the amount of moisture in a wound is crucial to the healing process. That's why dressings are commonly classified according to whether they add moisture to a wound bed or whether they absorb it.

Selecting the right dressing for a wound means taking into account:
- the size of the wound
- the amount of moisture in the wound
- whether the wound is infected
- the condition of the surrounding skin.

Dressing moisture scale

Use this chart to quickly determine the category of dressing that's appropriate for your patient.

Absorb moisture ← | **Neutral** (maintain existing moisture level) | → **Add moisture**

• Alginates/ fibers	• Foams	• Composites	• Transparent films	• Sheet hydrogels	• Amorphous hydrogels
• Gauze	• Wound fillers		• Hydrocolloids		• Hydrogel-impregnated gauze or gauze strips
			• Cellular tissue products		
			• Collagen dressings		
			• Contact layers		

Alginate/fiber dressings

Made from seaweed, alginate dressings are available as sterile pads, ribbons, or ropes. These nonocclusive dressings are nonadherent and promote autolytic debridement to soften and remove necrotic tissue. Fiber dressings are similar in appearance to alginates, absorb exudate, and lock in the exudate by forming a gel.

Alginate dressing in rope form

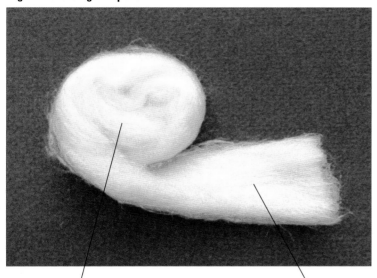

Very soft, nonwoven fibers turn into a biodegradable gel as they absorb exudate.

Fibers encourage hemostasis in minimally bleeding wounds.

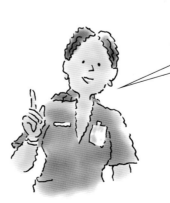

To facilitate dressing removal—and to make dressing changes less painful—saturate the dressing with normal saline solution before removal. Use additional saline to clean the wound of any remaining dressing fibers. If dressing is dry, consider the use of another wound dressing.

Antimicrobial dressings

Antimicrobial dressings contain ingredients such as silver, iodine, and polyhexamethylene to protect against bacteria. Available in various forms—including transparent dressings, gauze, island dressings, foams, and absorptive fillers—some antimicrobial dressings also provide a moist environment for wound healing.

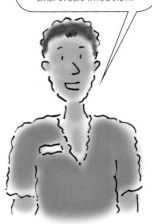

Silver has powerful antimicrobial and bactericidal properties. In fact, it's been used for centuries to prevent and treat infection.

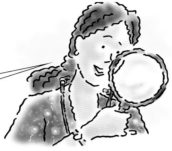

Silver in the dressing attacks bacteria and helps bind toxins.

Silver-impregnated antimicrobial dressing

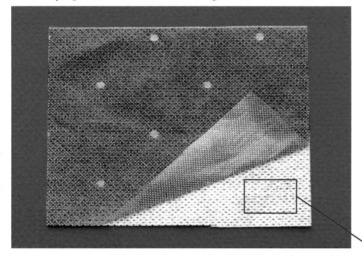

Silver-impregnated activated charcoal cloth

Silver ions

Bacteria

Bacteria leaking fluid as it dies

How antimicrobial dressings work

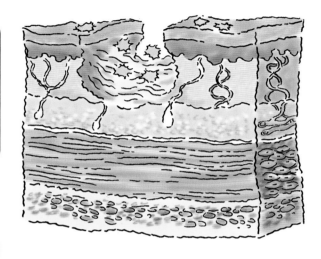

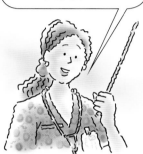

Signs of wound infection include redness, swelling, increased pain, and increased drainage. If that isn't bad enough, infection can stop the healing process and worsen wound breakdown.

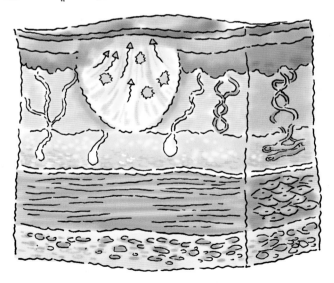

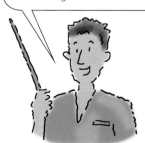

Once applied, some silver dressings immediately begin to release silver in a controlled fashion. The silver destroys bacteria in the dressing and the wound.

Collagen dressings

Made with bovine or avian collagen, collagen dressings are available in sheets, pads, particles, and gels.

Collagen dressings encourage wound healing by stimulating the deposit of collagen fibers necessary for the growth of tissue and blood vessels.

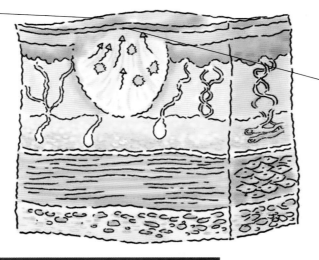

These highly absorbent dressings also maintain a moist wound environment.

Collagen in particle form

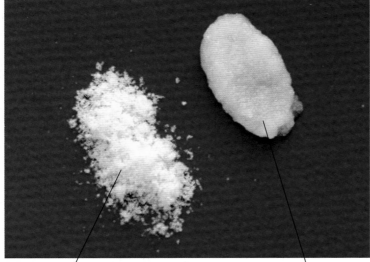

Some bovine collagen is processed into fine particles, as shown here. These particles can then be shaken into a wound bed.

Mixing with moist exudate in the wound, the particles gel as they absorb many times their weight in excess fluid.

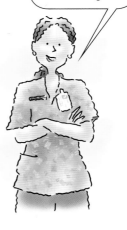

Make sure that wound infection has been treated and necrotic tissue debrided before using a collagen dressing.

Composite dressings

Composite dressings combine two or more types of dressings into one. Typical layers include:

1 Waterproof, vapor-permeable film

2 Absorbent foam layer

3 Silicone inner layer

> By combining two or more materials into one dressing, composite dressings reduce confusion and make dressing changes a snap.

SNAP

A closer look at a composite dressing

This composite dressing stimulates autolytic debridement while controlling moisture.

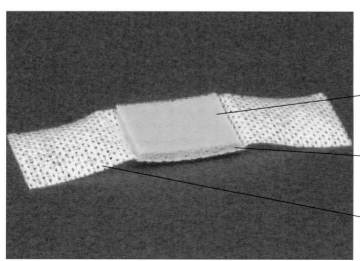

A thin, transparent, semipermeable film allows the exchange of gas and water vapor while blocking bacteria.

A highly absorbent foam-type matrix slowly releases ingredients that clean and moisturize the wound.

The adhesive backing consists of a breathable cloth.

Contact layer dressings

Made of woven or perforated material, contact layer dressings are single-layer dressings designed to lie directly on the wound's surface. A secondary dressing is then placed on top of the contact layer.

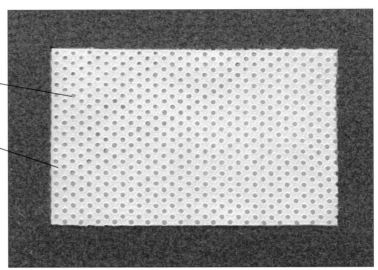

Holes allow drainage to pass through to a secondary dressing.

During dressing changes, the contact layer remains in place to protect the wound from trauma.

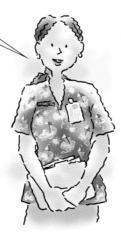

Contact layer dressings are usually made of silicone because of silicone's nonallergic and nonstick properties.

Fillers

Used to fill deep wounds, some wound fillers add moisture to the wound bed whereas others absorb drainage. Made of various materials, wound fillers are available as pastes, granules, strands, powders, beads, and gels.

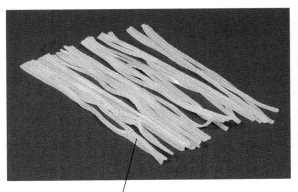

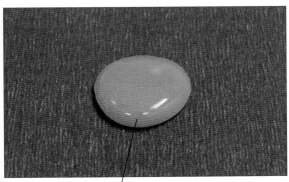

Wound filler in strand form

- Highly absorbent properties make it appropriate for wounds with heavy exudate.
- Strand form allows material to completely fill dead space.
- This particular filler contains silver, which has antimicrobial properties.

Wound filler in gel form

- Gel fills the wound evenly, helping prevent wound dehydration.
- Some gels effectively control wound odor.
- This dextrose-based gel mixes with wound drainage to coat and protect the wound and to provide a moist healing environment.

Foam dressings

Foam dressings are absorbent, spongelike polymer dressings. In addition to providing thermal insulation, they help maintain a moist wound environment while absorbing excess exudate.

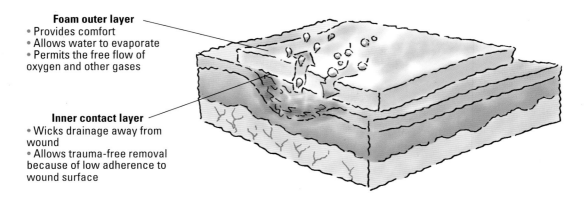

Foam outer layer
- Provides comfort
- Allows water to evaporate
- Permits the free flow of oxygen and other gases

Inner contact layer
- Wicks drainage away from wound
- Allows trauma-free removal because of low adherence to wound surface

Adhesive foam dressing

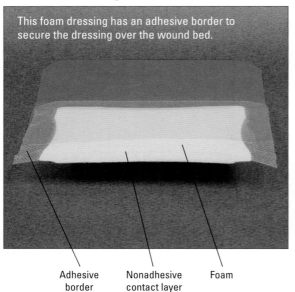

This foam dressing has an adhesive border to secure the dressing over the wound bed.

Adhesive border	Nonadhesive contact layer	Foam

Nonadhesive foam dressing

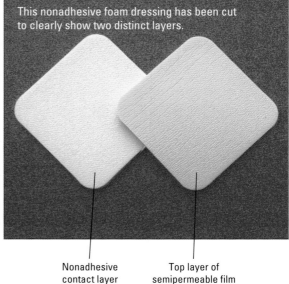

This nonadhesive foam dressing has been cut to clearly show two distinct layers.

Nonadhesive contact layer	Top layer of semipermeable film

Hydrocolloid dressings

Made of a carbohydrate-based material, hydrocolloid dressings are adhesive, moldable wafers that are impermeable to oxygen, water, and water vapor. Besides being somewhat absorbent, these dressings help maintain a moist wound environment and promote autolytic debridement. These dressings are available in various thicknesses.

> Hydrocolloids turn to gel as they absorb moisture, making the dressing become spongy and lighter in color over the wound. Reassure the patient that this is normal and, by itself, doesn't necessitate a dressing change.

Hydrocolloid dressing

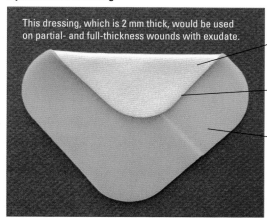

This dressing, which is 2 mm thick, would be used on partial- and full-thickness wounds with exudate.

The exterior surface protects the wound from outside contaminants.

The hydrocolloid layer turns to gel as hydrocolloids absorb moisture.

The adhesive layer adheres to the surrounding skin, but not the wound; adherence decreases as gel forms.

Thin hydrocolloid dressing

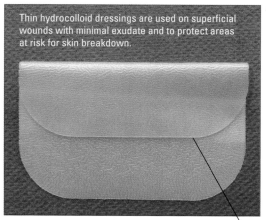

Thin hydrocolloid dressings are used on superficial wounds with minimal exudate and to protect areas at risk for skin breakdown.

The hydrocolloid interior of this dressing is less than 1 mm thick.

Hydrocolloid paste and gel

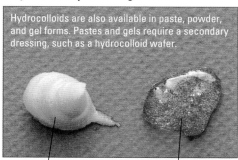

Hydrocolloids are also available in paste, powder, and gel forms. Pastes and gels require a secondary dressing, such as a hydrocolloid wafer.

Hydrocolloid paste
• Used to manage dermal wounds with light drainage

Hydrocolloid gel
• Used on partial- and full-thickness wounds
• Fills dry wound cavities
• Promotes autolytic debridement

Hydrogel dressings

Made with a water or glycerin base, hydrogel dressings hydrate wounds and soften necrotic tissue. Most contain a large percentage of water, and consequently these dressings provide limited absorption. Hydrogel dressings are available as a flexible sheet, impregnated gauze in pad or strip, or as an amorphous gel.

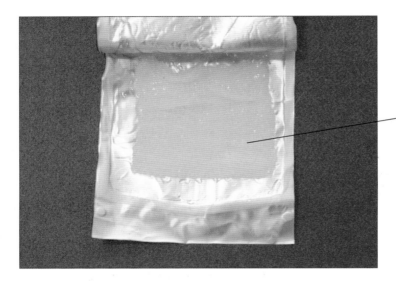

Hydrogel-impregnated gauze
- Hydrates wounds
- Softens necrotic tissue
- Cools and soothes burning wounds (such as skin tears and dermal wounds)

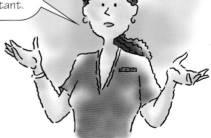

There's a good and bad side to every story. Although hydrogel dressings are great for hydrating wounds, they can also macerate the surrounding skin. Protect the healthy skin around the wound by fitting the dressing to the wound and applying a skin protectant.

Amorphous hydrogels

Amorphous hydrogels are gels packaged in tubes. Depending on the components in the gel, amorphous hydrogels have a number of uses.

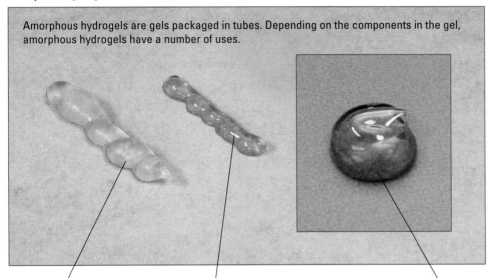

Plain hydrogel
• Creates a moist wound environment
• Promotes autolytic debridement

20% sodium chloride gel
• Increases the level of sodium in the wound bed
• Has an enhanced ability to soften and remove necrotic tissue

Hydrogel with additives (such as alginate)
• Absorbs low to moderate amounts of drainage

Transparent film dressings

Made of polyurethane, transparent film dressings adhere to the skin and help maintain a moist wound environment. While these dressings are nonabsorbent, they promote autolytic debridement and stimulate the formation of granulation tissue.

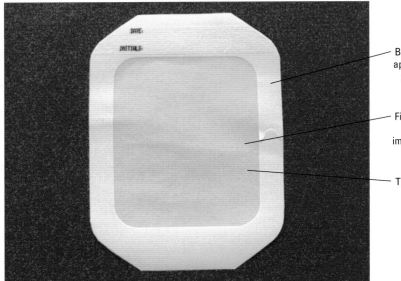

Backing is removed before application, leaving a clear, membranelike dressing.

Film allows the exchange of water vapor and oxygen while being impermeable to fluids and bacteria.

Transparent film allows visual inspection of the wound while the dressing is in place.

Wound care dressing review

Use this chart to quickly compare the various dressings, their actions, indications for use, contraindications, and dressing tips.

This chart contains dressing classifications with some actions, indications, contraindications, and application tips for the classifications.

Dressing Classifications	Actions	Indications	Contraindications	Application tip
Alginates/Fibers Pads or ropes	• Absorb drainage • Most fibers or alginates form a gel when they become wet	• Wounds with moderate to heavy drainage • Wounds with draining tunnels	• Dry wounds	• Keep fiber or alginate inside wound • Need an absorptive secondary dressing • Protect periwound skin with skin prep
Antimicrobials Silver Cadexomer Iodine Polyhexamethylene biguanide Honey	• Kill bacteria and reduce bioburden while remaining non-cytotoxic for wound healing and cell proliferation	• Infected wounds • Wounds suspected to have bioburden	• Allergy to product components	• See manufacturer directions • For honey, use only medical grade honey
Cellular Tissue Products (CTPs) *(Indications, contraindications, & application depend on type of CTP used)*	• Each product acts differently • Contain living or preserved animal or human tissue or cells important in wound healing	• Nonhealing diabetic foot ulcers, venous ulcers, pressure ulcers—check manufacturer directions	• If bovine product, check for allergy to bovine • Do not use on clinically infected wounds	• See manufacturer directions as there may be a specific way to handle certain CTPs
Collagen Dressings	• Provides collagen matrix to wound bed to accelerate wound healing	• To 'jump start' a wound that is not healing by providing a scaffold for cells to use to enhance healing	• Dry, eschar covered wounds • 3rd degree burns • Not most effective on necrotic wounds • If bovine product, check for allergy to bovine	• Select dressing based on wound bed • Use cover dressings as needed for absorbency, protection, etc. • Remove by rinsing wound with NSS and reapplying dressing material

Wound care dressing review *(continued)*

Dressing Classifications	Actions	Indications	Contraindications	Application tip
Composites	• Hybrid dressings combining two or more types of dressings	• Minimal to moderate absorptive capability • Partial to full thickness • Clean or necrotic	• May dry out wound bed depending on product selected • Cannot be cut to fit without losing integrity • Do not use on 3rd degree burns	• Consider skin prep on periwound skin
Contact Layers Nonadherent dressings	• Minimal absorptive capability • Nonstick surface	• Helps prevent dressing adherence • Helps protect regenerating tissue and minimizes patient pain and trauma during dressing changes • Exudate easily passes through to the secondary absorbent dressing or to negative pressure wound therapy • Can be cut to wound size without unraveling and shredding	• Heavily exudative wounds unless you are using the dressing as a wound contact layer under NPWT • 3rd degree burns	• Consider skin prep on periwound skin

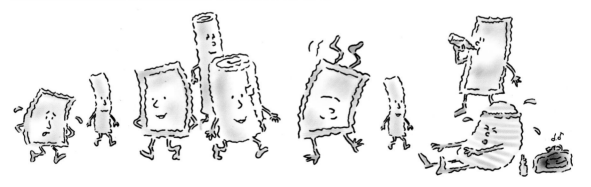

Wound care dressing review *(continued)*

Dressing Classifications	Actions	Indications	Contraindications	Application tip
Fillers	• Fill deeper wounds, tracts/tunnels, under-mined areas • Add moisture or absorb depending on product selected	• Dead space in wound	• Some dressings cannot be used on burns or wounds with little or no drainage	• Follow manufacturer's directions for application and removal
Foams	• Absorbs exudate and holds exudate away from wound bed • Permits moist environment without maceration	• Assists with autolytic debridement of moist wound bed • Absorbs moderate to heavy exudate • Insulates wound surface • May provide nontrau-matic removal • Partial thickness • Full thickness if dead space is lightly filled • May be used as a secondary dressing for additional absorption • Clean or dirty wounds	• Wounds with no exudate (some foams are not as hydrophilic as others and may be used with drier wounds) • Wounds with dry eschar • Wounds with undermining edges or sinus tracts unless areas are lightly filled	• Foam needs to be secured if it is nonadhe-sive (tape, gauze wrap, mesh net wrap, elastic bandage) • Use skin protectant around wound to protect from drainage • Change when drainage strikes through to outer edges of foam (or top of foam depending on product) Q 2 to 5 days

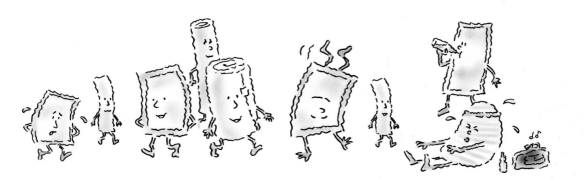

Wound care dressing review *(continued)*

Dressing Classifications	Actions	Indications	Contraindications	Application tip
Gauze "Gauze" dressings were traditionally woven cotton, nonfilled, sponges that may be loosely woven or a fine mesh. 2×2 and 4×4 are most common sizes **Noncotton, nonwoven** Synthetic gauze is now available in several combinations, polyester and/or rayon	• Absorbs exudate and allows fluid to transfer to secondary dressing; nonselective debridement of wound bed; fills dead space of wound, sinus tract/ tunnel, or undermining edges • Absorbent but does not transfer drainage to secondary dressing as well as cotton gauze	• Gauze dressings are used on all wound stages • Most effective on full thickness but should to be changed Q 4-8 hrs, to maintain moisture	• Lightly filled in dry wounds unless moistened	• Fine mesh gauze to ↓ damage to wound bed on removal (do not use cotton-filled sponges as 'debris' can be left in wound) • Fill lightly to avoid compromised blood flow or delay wound closure • Protect surrounding skin with a skin protector when moist gauze used or wound is draining • Change Q 4 to 8 hrs, depending on purpose, amt. of drainage • For draining wound, use cotton gauze to "wick" drainage into secondary dressing (such as an ABD)

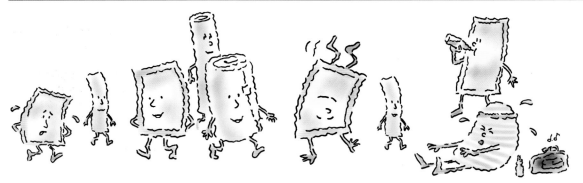

Wound care dressing review *(continued)*

Dressing Classifications	Actions	Indications	Contraindications	Application tip
Hydrocolloids	• Contains hydroactive particles • Occlusive • May react with wound exudate to form gel-like covering to maintain moist wound environment • Absorbs low to moderate amount of exudate	• Assists with autolytic debridement by keeping wound bed moist • Absorbs light to moderate wound drainage • Insulates wound and because of occlusion provides some protection against secondary infection • Partial thickness • Shallow full thickness (think ear) • Noninfected wounds	• Highly exudative wounds • Clinically infected wounds • Wounds with sinus tracts/tunnels or undermining edges unless this "dead space" is lightly filled	• 1 1/2 to 2 inches of intact skin around wound allows for better seal • May use skin protector around wound to defat area and protect skin from adhesive if fragile skin — Check manufacturer's directions • Shave or clip excessive hair to ↓ bacterial invasion of wound and ↑ adhesion • "Picture frame edges with tape if dressing not prepackaged with this feature • Change Q 3 days or when dressing is no longer occlusive, leaking, or wrinkled • Exudate is usually yellowish and odorous—assess wound **after** cleaning • Does not require secondary dressing • Occlusive so stool and urine do not contaminate wound unless dressing is not intact

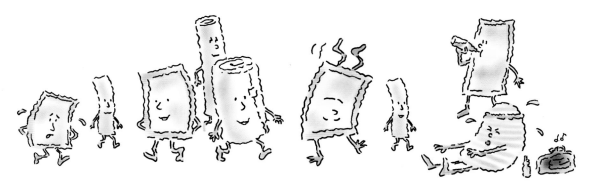

Wound care dressing review *(continued)*

Dressing Classifications	Actions	Indications	Contraindications	Application tip

Hydrogel sheet dressing
 	
Amorphous wound gel
 	
Hydrogel-impregnated gauze pads and gauze strips
	• Maintain a moist wound surface as they are composed of mostly water
	• Nonadherent
	• Minimal absorption
	• Autolytic debridement because of eschar hydration
	• Sheet acts like second layer of skin and decreases pain
	• Amorphous gels have different hydrophilic properties and therefore have different wound hydrating capacities—check product info.
		• Promote autolytic debridement
		• Provides comfort to wound
		• Clean or dirty
		• Partial thickness
		  – Sheet—Cut to fit wound as moist dressing can macerate intact skin around the wound
		  – Amorphous—Consider using nonabsorptive dressing to decrease amount of wound gel absorbed by secondary dressing
		• Filling dead space
		  – Amorphous—Use NSS moistened gauze, fluffed, to fill dead space after gel applied to wound surface
		  – Use manufactured, impregnated gel gauze to fill dead space…still fluff the gauze
		  – Strip gauze for tracts/tunnels
			• Moderate to heavily exudative wounds	• Secondary dressings are needed
				• Change dressings when strike through occurs; may be once or twice a day to every other day

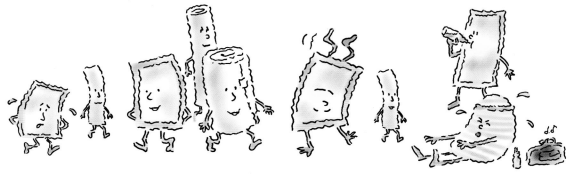

Wound care dressing review *(continued)*

Dressing Classifications	Actions	Indications	Contraindications	Application tip
Transparent, polyurethane adhesive film	• Semipermeable membrane that permits water vapor and oxygen to pass between wound bed and environment but keeps bacteria from coming in because of dressing pore size • Maintains moist wound environment to enhance resurfacing of the wound • Occlusion reduces local wound pain • Autolytic debridement enhanced by moist, warm environment • Does not require secondary dressing	• Indicated for non-draining wounds. Supports autolytic debridement of dry eschar and fibrin slough • Maintains moist, non-adherent surface next to wound • Protects blisters and superficial wounds easily • Wound can be monitored through transparent dressing • Partial thickness • Do not use on infected wounds • May be used as secondary dressing for selected wounds	• Exudative wounds. Clinically infected wounds • Wounds with sinus tracts or undermining edges unless this "dead space" is lightly filled	• 1 1/2 to 2 inches of intact skin around wound allows for better seal • Use skin protector around wound to defat area and protect skin from adhesive • Shave or clip excessive hair to ↓ bacterial invasion of wound & ↑ adhesion • Change when dressing is leaking or no longer intact or Q 3 to 5 days • Exudate is usually cloudy and foul smelling until wound cleansed

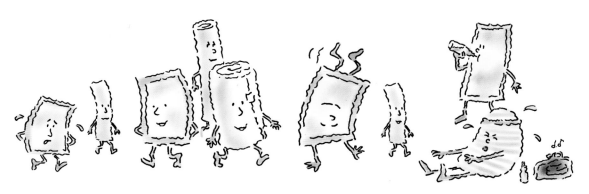

Other treatments

Topical drugs and other treatments can complement the function of dressings to promote wound healing.

Debriding agents

Enzyme preparations called *debriding agents* are topically applied to necrotic or devitalized tissue to help facilitate its removal from a wound. Follow the manufacturer's directions for amount to be applied.

Crosshatching helps to ensure that the debriding agent penetrates the tissue so that it can begin to liquefy and digest necrotic tissue.

Necrotic tissue

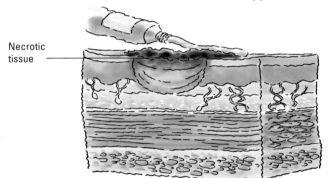

1

First, apply the debriding agent to the surface of the wound after crosshatching any eschar (scoring it with a scalpel in a meshlike pattern), taking care to apply to entire wound bed per manufacturer recommendations.

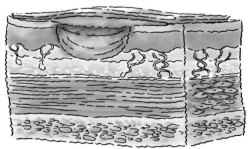

2

Apply damp NSS dressing over ointment and then cover with dry dressing

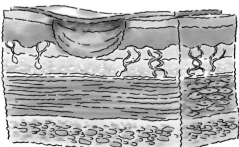

3

Once daily, remove the dressing and irrigate the wound to remove the liquefied necrotic material. Afterward, apply more debriding agent and a clean dressing.

Negative pressure wound therapy

When a wound fails to heal in a timely manner, negative pressure wound therapy (NPWT) may be used.

The dressing used with NPWT devices varies, depending upon the wound being treated, as well as the NPWT system used. Some systems use gauze to fill the wound, others use foam. In addition, disposable units are now available for incision care or for wounds with minimal drainage. When turned on, the pump gently reduces air pressure beneath the dressing, drawing off exudate and reducing edema in surrounding tissues. This process reduces bacterial colonization, promotes granulation tissue development, increases the rate of cell mitosis, and spurs the migration of epithelial cells within the wound.

A denser white foam dressing is available and the purpose of this dressing is to reduce the growth of granulation tissue into the dressing (which reduces the pain of dressing changes), protect delicate structures, and prevent wound adherence.

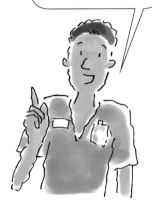

> Choosing which dressing to use with NPWT isn't always a black or white issue. Some systems may use a gauze dressing.

Black Foam dressing

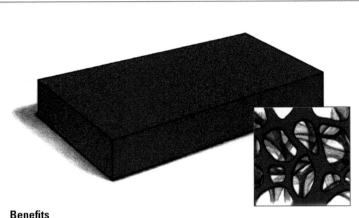

Benefits
The open, porous structure of this polyurethane dressing:
- stimulates the formation of granulation tissue
- evenly distributes negative pressure throughout the wound
- facilitates the removal of drainage.

Indications
- Deep acute wounds
- Deep pressure injuries
- Flaps

White foam dressing

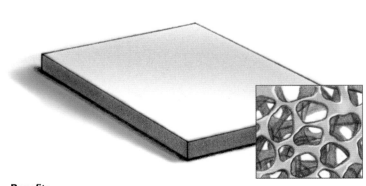

Benefits
This dense dressing made of a microporous polyvinyl alcohol material:
- reduces the growth of granulation tissue into the dressing (which reduces the pain of dressing changes)
- protects delicate structures
- prevents wound adherence.

Indications
- Wounds with sufficient granulation tissue
- Wounds with exposed muscle, tendons, bone
- Wounds with tunnels, sinus tracts, or areas of undermining
- Superficial wounds
- Painful wounds
Incisions

Applying tNPWT dressing

3

Apply the pad with tubing over the hole made in the drape.

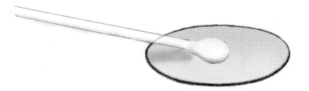

2

Cut the drape to extend 1¼′ to 2′ (3 to 5 cm) over adjacent skin in all directions. Make a small hole in the center. Seal the drape securely.

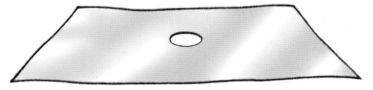

1

Cut the foam dressing to fit the size and shape of the wound, extending it into areas of tunneling or undermining.

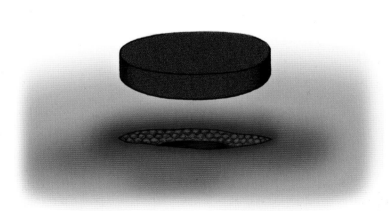

Growth factor therapy

Growth factor therapy is a type of biotherapy used to stimulate cell proliferation in wound treatment. The growth factor must be synthesized, secreted, and removed from the tissues at the correct time to prevent stalling of wound healing. It should be applied using a sterile applicator, such as a swab or tongue blade, or saline-moistened gauze. Then the wound should be dressed with saline-moistened gauze. It should not be used on an infected wound.

Hyperbaric oxygen therapy

Hyperbaric oxygen therapy involves the delivery of 100% oxygen to a patient in a sealed chamber. A total body chamber increases the amount of dissolved oxygen in the blood that's available for wound healing.

Hyperbaric oxygen chamber

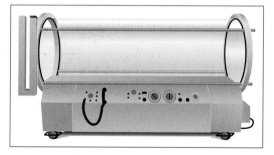

Understanding growth factors

Type	Description
TGF-β (transforming growth factor beta)	Controls movement of cells to sites of inflammation and stimulates extracellular matrix formation
bFGF (basic fibroblast growth factor)	Stimulates angiogenesis (the development of blood vessels)
VEGF (vascular endothelial growth factor)	Stimulates angiogenesis
IGF (insulin-like growth factor)	Increases collagen synthesis
EGF (epidermal growth factor)	Stimulates epidermal regeneration

Pulsatile lavage

Pulsatile lavage is a form of hydrotherapy that can be used with almost any wound type. It involves the application of room temperature sterile normal saline solution to the wound bed under pressure using a spray gun with simultaneous aspiration of the solution by negative pressure through a separate tube in the gun.

Pulsatile lavage gun

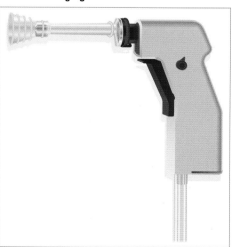

Ultraviolet radiation therapy

Ultraviolet (UV) radiation therapy is used to treat slowly healing wounds, necrotic wounds, and infected or heavily contaminated wounds.

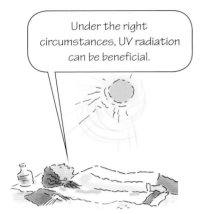

Under the right circumstances, UV radiation can be beneficial.

UVC radiation device

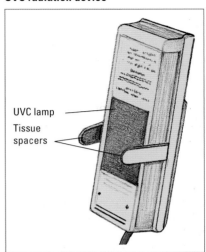

UVC lamp

Tissue spacers

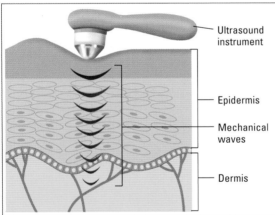

Ultrasound instrument

Epidermis

Mechanical waves

Dermis

Ultrasound treatment

In ultrasound treatment, mechanical pressure waves are used to hasten healing and help decrease pain and inflammation. Optimal effects are seen when this treatment is used during the inflammatory phase of wound healing.

Electrical stimulation device

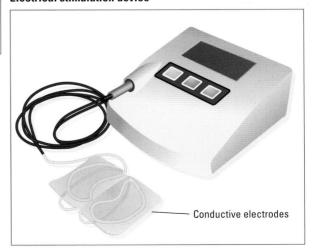

Conductive electrodes

Electrical stimulation treatment

In electrical stimulation, electrical current is delivered by conductive electrodes to the skin or to the skin and a wound to enhance healing.

Review of other wound care treatments

Use this chart to quickly review the indications for use, advantages, and disadvantages of other wound care treatments.

Drug or device	Indications for use	Advantages	Disadvantages
Debriding agent (only agent is Collagenase SANTYL)	• Wounds with moderate to large amounts of necrotic tissue • Wounds in which surgical debridement is contraindicated	• Effective alternative to surgical or sharp debridement	• Requires secondary dressings • May irritate surrounding skin • Not compatible with iodine and many silver products
Negative pressure wound therapy	• Slow-healing acute, subacute, or chronic exudative wounds with cavities • Pressure injuries or surgical wounds more than 1 cm deep To stabilize new grafts Surgical incisions	• Cleans deeply and can manage moderate to large amounts of drainage • Can manage multiple wounds when dressings are cut to bridge two or more wounds • May allow patient mobility (some models have rechargeable batteries and are small enough to fit in a pouch worn at the waist or over the shoulder)	• Is contraindicated for untreated osteomyelitis, malignancies, and wounds with necrotic tissue or fistulas • May require electricity or rechargeable batteries to operate • Be alert for excessive bloody drainage
Becaplermin growth factor therapy —Example: Platelet-derived growth factor becaplermin (Regranex)	• Full-thickness diabetic neuropathic ulcers that have adequate blood flow • Clean, noninfected, granulating wounds	• Provides growth factors needed for wound healing • Attracts fibroblasts and induces them to divide, which aids wound healing • Must be applied only once daily • Requires no special training for application	• Can't be used on necrotic tissue or infected wounds • Is contraindicated in patients with poor blood supply to the legs or neoplasms near the wound • May cause a localized rash
Hyperbaric oxygen therapy	• If wounds have not improved with traditional therapies, HBO for diabetic foot ulcers, osteoradionecrosis, and selected other chronic wounds may be helpful.	• Enhances the activity of neutrophils • Relieves relative hypoxia in wound tissues	• Is contraindicated in patients taking antineoplastic agents and those with known pneumothorax
Pulsatile lavage	• Infected or heavily contaminated wounds • Wounds that require preparation for grafting with either skin grafts or living skin equivalents • Wounds that require removal of necrotic tissue or other particulate matter	• Increases granulation tissue formation in clean and slow-healing wounds • Decreases bioburden levels in infected or heavily contaminated wounds • Is less uncomfortable than some other treatments • Is easily accessible due to portability of the equipment • Is effective in reaching deep, tunneling wounds • Minimizes cross contamination	• Requires the use of low impact and suction pressure on fragile tissue and avoiding direct pressure over exposed nerves and blood vessels

Review of other wound care treatments *(continued)*

Drug or device	Indications for use	Advantages	Disadvantages
Ultraviolet radiation therapy	• Chronic, slow healing wounds • Infected or heavily contaminated wounds • Necrotic wounds	*UVA and UVB radiation* • Increases wound healing in chronic pressure ulcers • Enhances white blood cell (WBC) accumulation and lysosomal activity in wounds • Increases production of interleukin-1 alpha (a cytokine involved in epithelialization) *UVC radiation* • Kills a broad spectrum of microorganisms with low exposure times • Is quickly and easily administered	• Is contraindicated in patients with a history of skin cancer, diabetes, pulmonary tuberculosis, hyperthyroidism, systemic lupus erythematosus, acute eczema, herpes simplex, or cardiac, renal, or hepatic disease
Ultrasound treatment	• Open and closed wounds	• Is portable • Requires only a short application time • Doesn't require dependent positioning • Involves no risk of maceration • Reduces bioburden • Increases WBC migration to the wound bed • Promotes orderly arrangement of collagen in wounds	• May require several treatment sessions (for large wounds) • May be painful or difficult to apply over irregular surfaces • Increases the risk of wound contamination
Electrical stimulation	• Recalcitrant wounds, especially chronic pressure ulcers	• Promotes cellular migration • Enhances blood flow • Increases protein synthesis and wound bed formation • Destroys microorganisms • Increases angiogenesis and tissue oxygenation • Reduces wound bioburden, microbial content, and wound and diabetic neuropathic pain	• Can't be used on malignant tissue • Can't be used over the pericardial area, other areas related to control of cardiac and respiratory function, or implanted devices • Is contraindicated in patients with untreated osteomyelitis

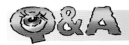

My word!

Use the clues to help you unscramble the names of three types of wound dressings. Then use the circled letters to answer the question posed.

Question: Controlling the amount of moisture in a wound is crucial for what to occur?

1. These dressings contain multiple layers of highly absorbent material, such as cotton or rayon.

   spaceylit vaporsbite

   — — ◯ — — — ◯ — — — ◯ — — — — — — — — —

2. Made from seaweed, these dressings contain very soft, nonwoven fibers that turn into a biodegradable gel as they absorb exudate.

   alientag   — — ◯ — ◯ — — —

3. These adhesive, moldable wafers are impermeable to oxygen, water, and water vapor.

   coldhydrooil   ◯ — — — — — — — — — — ◯ —

Answer: — — — — — — —

Show and tell

Describe the steps for applying a debriding agent to a wound based on the images shown.

1. _____

_____

_____

_____

2. _____

_____

_____

_____

3. _____

_____

_____

_____

Selected References

Broussard, K. C., & Powers, J. G. (2013). Wound dressings: Selecting the most appropriate type..*American Journal Clinical Dermatology, 14*(6), 449–459.

Doughty, D., & McNichol, L. (Eds.) (2016). *Wound Ostomy and Continence Nurses Society Core Curriculum Wound Management*. Philadelphia, PA: Wolters Kluwer.

Doughty, D., & McNichol, L. (2016). Wound, Ostomy, and Continence Nurses Society Core Curriculum: Wound management. WOCN.

Haesler, E., & White, W. (2017). Minimising wound-related pain: A discussion of traditional wound dressings and topical agents used in low-resource communities. *Wound Practice and Research, 25*(3), 138–144.

National Pressure Ulcer Advisory Panel, European Pressure Ulcer Advisory Panel, and Pan Pacific Pressure Injury Alliance. (2014). *Prevention and treatment of pressure ulcers: Clinical practice guideline*. Osborne Park, Western Australia: Cambridge Media.

Robbins, J. M., & Dillon, J. (2015). Evidence-based approach to advanced wound care products. *Journal of the American Podiatric Medical Association, 105*(5), 456–467. doi:10.7547/14-089

Index